DASH DIET CO FOR BEGINNERS

Banish Health Worries and Achieve Weight Loss with 1500 Days of Family-Approved, Quick, and Delicious Low-Sodium Recipes- Guide to Lower Blood Pressure, Live Healthier

Maya Green

Copyright 2023 All Rights Reserved

Legal Disclaimer
This book, "Dash Diet Cookbook for Beginners," is protected by copyright laws. No part of this publication may be reproduced or transmitted in any form without the prior written permission of the author.

Disclaimer Notice
The information provided in this book is intended for recreational purposes only. It is not intended to replace professional medical advice, diagnosis, or treatment. The content of this book is based on research and personal experiences, and it is not written by medical professionals. Therefore, it is strongly recommended that you consult with your healthcare provider and a qualified professional before implementing any advice or recommendations presented in this book.
Each individual's health situation is unique, and the Dash Diet may not be suitable for everyone. Your healthcare provider can evaluate your specific health condition and provide personalized guidance. They can help you determine if the Dash Diet is appropriate for you and assist in tailoring it to meet your specific needs and goals.

The author and publisher of this book are not responsible for any adverse effects or consequences resulting from the use of the information provided. The reader assumes full responsibility for their actions and decisions based on the content of this book.
By reading this book, you acknowledge that you have read and understood the above disclaimer.

Table of Contents

INTRODUCTION 5
  DASH Diet Fundamentals and Benefits 5
    What is Dash Diet? 5
    Benefits of Dash Diet 6
  Food Guidelines 7
    Not Recommended for Dash Diet Food List 9
    Role of Salt 10
    Recommended Daily Limits 11
  Shopping List 12
  DASH Diet Success Stories 14

CHAPTER 1. BREAKFAST RECIPES 16
  1. Breakfast Omelet 16
  2. Triple Berry Steel Cut Oats 16
  3. Breakfast Porridge 16
  4. Coconut Almond Granola 17
  5. Breakfast Oatmeal 17
  6. Tomato Omelet 17
  7. Breakfast Eggnog 18
  8. Slow Cooker French Toast Casserole 18
  9. Apple Cinnamon Steel Cut Oats 18
  10. Breakfast Casserole 19
  11. Chia Breakfast Pudding 19
  12. Breakfast Stuffed Biscuits 19
  13. Ground Beef Breakfast Skillet 19
  14. Pumpkin Quinoa Porridge 20
  15. Gingerbread Oatmeal 20
  16. Maple Oatmeal 20
  17. Banana Chia Pudding 21
  18. Breakfast Tofu 21
  19. At-Home Cappuccino 22
  20. Blueberry Low-Sodium Pancakes 22
  21. Barley Porridge 22
  22. Breakfast Frittata 23
  23. Apples and Cinnamon Oatmeal 23
  24. Apple Oats 23
  25. Breakfast Rice Porridge 23

CHAPTER 2. RECIPES FOR LUNCHES 25
  26. Pork with Scallions and Peanuts 25
  27. Creamy Smoky Pork Chops 25
  28. Southwestern Chicken and Pasta 25
  29. Spiced Winter Pork Roast 26
  30. Pork Chops And Apples 26
  31. Shrimp with Garlic and Mushrooms 26
  32. Thai Curry with Prawns 27
  33. Ginger And Chili Baked Fish 27

  34. Beef Stroganoff 28
  35. Chicken Veronique 28
  36. Chicken Chili 29
  37. Mediterranean Fish Bake 29
  38. Baked Salmon 30
  39. Healthy, Juicy Salmon Dish 30
  40. Sesame Salmon With Broccoli And Tomatoes 31
  41. Mediterranean Pork 31
  42. Tuna and Potato Bake 32
  43. Mussels with Tomatoes & Chili 32
  44. Currant Pork Chops 32
  45. Chicken Divan 33
  46. Crunchy Fish Bites 33
  47. Mediterranean Beef Dish 34
  48. Smoked Salmon Crudités 34
  49. Balsamic-Roasted Chicken Breasts 34
  50. Sesame Chicken Veggie Wraps 35

CHAPTER 3. RECIPES FOR DINNERS 36
  51. Chicken Tomato and Green Beans 36
  52. Pork Strips and Rice 36
  53. Fish with Peppers 36
  54. Taco-Seasoned Roast Beef Wraps 37
  55. Seafood Risotto 37
  56. Chicken & Goat Cheese Skillet 38
  57. Lamb Chops With Minted Peas And Feta 38
  58. Prawn Nasi Goreng 39
  59. Steak Tuna 39
  60. Pork and Sweet Potatoes 39
  61. Lemon-Parsley Chicken Breast 40
  62. Grilled Salmon With Papaya-Mint Salsa 40
  63. Pork and Pumpkin Chili 41
  64. Pumpkin and Black Beans Chicken 41
  65. Lemon Rosemary Branzino 41
  66. Spicy Chicken with Minty Couscous 42
  67. Mussels With Creamy Tarragon Sauce 42
  68. Pesto Chicken Breasts 43
  69. Pork and Veggies Mix 43
  70. Spiced Up Pork Chops 44
  71. Herbed Butter Pork Chops 44
  72. Pork With Dates Sauce 45
  73. Ground Beef and Bell Peppers 45
  74. Cilantro Lemon Shrimp 45
  75. Parsley Scallops 46

CHAPTER 4. RECIPES FOR SALADS AND SAUCES 47
  76. Pork and Greens Salad 47
  77. Garlic Potato Salad 47

78. Tomato-Basil Sauce	47
79. Tomato, Cucumber, and Basil Salad	48
80. Warm Potato Salad with Spinach	48
81. Chicken BBQ Salad	49
82. Sweet Potato Salad with Maple Vinaigrette	49
83. Zucchini-Ribbon Salad	50
84. Tart Apple Salad with Yogurt and Honey Dressing	50
85. Mexican Vegetable Salad	50
86. Fresh Herb Sauce	51
87. Spicy Avocado Sauce	51
88. Egg Salad	51
89. Chipotle Chicken Salad	52
90. Eggplant Salad	52
91. Cilantro-Lime Sauce	52
92. Strawberry Spinach Salad	53
93. Mandarin Salad	53
94. Lemon-Dill Yogurt Sauce	54
95. Mayo-Less Tuna Salad	54
96. Tropical Chicken Salad	54
97. Summer Corn Salad with Peppers and Avocado	55
98. Roasted Corn & Edamame Salad	55
99. Balsamic Glaze	56
100. Simple Autumn Salad	56

CHAPTER 5. RECIPES FOR SNACKS 57

101. Mango Salsa Wontons	57
102. Cauliflower And Leeks	57
103. Sweet and Spicy Kettle Corn	57
104. Eggplant And Mushroom Sauté	58
105. Mexican Layer Dip	58
106. Spicy Sweet Potatoes	58
107. Asparagus Bruschetta With Garlic And Basil	59
108. Hot Crab Dip	59
109. Mint Zucchini	60
110. Sweet And Spicy Meatballs	60
111. Broccoli And Almonds Mix	60
112. Fresh Tzatziki	61
113. Squash And Cranberries	61
114. Roasted Brussels Sprouts	61
115. Dill Carrots	62
116. Spicy Kale Chips	62
117. Cheese Herb Dip	63
118. Cinnamon Tortillas Chips	63
119. Grilled Sweet Potatoes And Scallions	63
120. Grilled Asparagus With Mozzarella	64
121. Celery And Kale Mix	64
122. Five Spice Chicken Lettuce Wraps	64
123. Warm Potato And Kale Mix	65
124. Kale, Mushrooms, And Red Chard Mix	65
125. Grilled Vegetables	66

CHAPTER 6. RECIPES FOR CAKES AND DESSERTS 67

126. Stone Cobbler	67
127. Banana Cookies	67
128. Apple Crunch Pie	68
129. Healthy Protein Bars	68
130. Strawberry Pie	68
131. Pineapple Meringues	69
132. Pound Cake with Pineapple	69
133. Mint Banana Chocolate Sorbet	69
134. Fudgesicles	70
135. Simple Apple Compote	70
136. Cocoa Fat Bombs	70
137. Light Pumpkin Pie Recipe	71
138. Stuffed Baked Apples	71
139. Almond and Tahini Cookies	71
140. Peanut Butter and Chocolate Balls	72
141. Almond Bites	72
142. Baked Egg Custard	73
143. Walnut Oatmeal Chocolate Chip Cookie	73
144. Sweet Raspberry Candy	74
145. Raspberry Yogurt Basted Cantaloupe	74
146. Dark Chocolate Trifle	74
147. Rhubarb Cake	75
148. Baba Ghanoush	75
149. Baked Custard	76
150. Peanut Butter Fat Bombs	76

CHAPTER 7. BONUS: DIET OBSTACLES AND VARIOUS SOLUTIONS 77

Meal Planning	77
Healthy Alternatives	77
Preventing Hunger Attacks	78
Reading Labels and Selecting Suitable Foods	78
Organizing the Pantry	78
Preparing Food in Advance	79
Social and Emotional Obstacles	79

30-DAY MEAL PLAN 80

MEASUREMENT CONVERSION CHART 82

RECIPE INDEX 84

CONCLUSION 86

Introduction

When it comes to changing your diet, the initial transition can often be the most challenging part. You will be able to eventually lose those excess lbs while making substantial progress towards enhancing your overall health if you develop an improved understanding of healthy food and monitor your calorie consumption. Recent years have seen an increase in the number of individuals with conditions such as high blood pressure, excess body fat, heart disease, and other ailments. The Dash Diet cookbook provides a perfect solution by incorporating a variety of healthy fruits, vegetables, and lean meats into your meals.

Also known as the Dietary Approaches to Stop Hypertension, the Dash Diet is a low-sodium eating plan that emphasizes the consumption of fruits and vegetables. It is one of the few diet plans that has been scientifically proven to effectively lower blood pressure. The underlying principle is that the majority of disease-causing inflammation in the body originates from our diet, as many diseases are associated with chronic inflammation. The Dash Diet focuses on adopting an anti-inflammatory lifestyle and aims to establish healthy eating habits that ultimately contribute to overall well-being.

By following the Dash Diet, you can lower your blood pressure, lose weight and lower the risk of various health problems such as heart disease, cancer, diabetes, and even dementia. The meals not only taste delicious but are also packed with essential vitamins and minerals necessary for a healthy body.

Unlike other diets that primarily focus on food restrictions, the Dash Diet promotes a dietary pattern that fosters a healthy lifestyle. This involves consuming ample amounts of fruits and vegetables, which helps limit the intake of inflammatory foods. The idea is to eliminate refined foods from your diet and replace them with options that are high in fibre, such as fruits and vegetables. Numerous studies have established that the Dash Diet significantly reduces blood pressure (up to 10 points) and aids in weight loss and lowering LDL ("bad") cholesterol. That's why the American Heart Association recommends it.

Adopting a healthy and balanced diet may not always be easy, but the Dash Diet can help you attain your health goals with its simple and convenient recipes. You can prepare delicious dishes for the entire family without spending excessive time in the kitchen.

By embracing the Dash Diet as a way of life, you will take essential steps towards eliminating active inflammation and preventing future diseases. Your energy levels will increase & you will experience an overall sense of well-being as your body becomes healthier each day. Start your new healthy lifestyle journey with the Dash Diet, and enjoy the numerous benefits it offers.

DASH Diet Fundamentals and Benefits

What is Dash Diet?

When contrasted with a low-fat diet, the Dash diet has been demonstrated to be over two and a half times more successful in bringing down the patient's blood pressure. It follows the "Load and Offset" philosophy, in which you fill your plate with whole grains, veggies, and nutritious proteins for six days out of the week, after which you fast for one day. Taking this strategy makes it easier to keep a healthy metabolic rate whilst also helping to keep blood pressure within control. The DASH study provided the basis for the diet's tenets, which were derived from the findings of a protracted piece of research.

The National Heart, Lung, and Blood Institute came up with the Dash diet with the intention of reducing the risk of cardiovascular disease and high blood pressure. It is estimated that 90% of Americans have undiagnosed hypertension, also known as the "silent killer" due to its lack of obvious symptoms until damage to the cardiovascular system occurs.

The Dash diet focuses on lowering sodium intake while promoting foods high in potassium, calcium, magnesium, and vitamins A, C, and E. Researchers believe that high sodium levels in our diets contribute to hypertension, raising blood pressure and increasing the risk of heart disease and stroke over time.

The Dash diet is based on two principles: a low-salt, balanced diet rich in fruits and vegetables, with a moderate amount of lean protein and no more than thirty percent of total daily calories from saturated fat, and regular physical activity to support cardiovascular health. It recommends limiting sodium intake to 2,300 mg per day or less for overall well-being.

By reducing sodium intake and increasing intake of potassium, calcium, and magnesium, the Dash diet can help lower blood pressure. Following this diet for two or more years can result in an average reduction of 5 mm Hg systolic and 2 mm Hg diastolic blood pressure. Lowering sodium intake has been found to have a greater impact on reducing systolic blood pressure than lowering saturated or total fat intake.

Not only does the Dash diet lower blood pressure, it may also have positive effects on sleep and mental health. Clinical trials have shown that compared to a diet lower in potassium and phosphorus, the Dash diet improves delta sleep scores and quality of life in individuals with hypertension.

Initially recommended for patients already on high blood pressure medications, the Dash diet has gained popularity as a means to lower blood pressure among healthy individuals. It can be administered in various ways, commonly as part of a weight loss plan due to its association with low-calorie diets. Some people follow the Dash diet solely to lower blood pressure, while others utilize it for weight loss, improved mental health & better sleep quality.

Benefits of Dash Diet

The Dash Diet offers a straightforward and effective approach to enhancing overall health and achieving weight loss. It focuses on incorporating fresh vegetables, fruits, whole grains, lean meats, and low-fat dairy products. The benefits of the Dash Diet are numerous:

1. **Healthy Weight Loss:** Research indicates that adopting a healthy eating pattern is key to successful weight loss. The Dash Diet has been proven to aid in weight reduction, lower blood pressure in obese individuals, and improve cholesterol levels. By providing fewer calories while still delivering essential nutrients, this diet promotes effective weight loss while supporting overall health.
2. **Improved Cholesterol Levels:** The Dash Diet is effective in reducing total blood cholesterol levels by approximately 1%. Studies demonstrate that closely adhering to this diet plan yields even greater improvements. By following the Dash Diet, individuals can lower LDL (bad) cholesterol levels & raise HDL (good) cholesterol levels more effectively than with a typical American diet. Lowering high blood pressure & improving cholesterol levels contribute to preventing and managing heart disease.
3. **Weight Loss:** It has been shown that the Dash Diet plays an important role in the weight loss. A study revealed that participants who adopted a healthy eating pattern and engaged in regular exercise experienced weight loss and reduced their risk of heart disease. Healthy eating, including reducing caloric intake and increasing physical activity, plays a crucial role in successful weight management.

4. **Improved Blood Pressure:** The Dash Diet is effective in lowering blood pressure in individuals with hypertension and pre-hypertension. Adopting a healthy eating pattern not only helps lower blood pressure but additionally averts heart disease and stroke. This diet is recommended for individuals with high blood pressure, pregnant women, diabetics, and those at risk of developing high blood pressure.
5. **Improved Blood Sugar Levels:** The Dash Diet promotes better blood sugar control by incorporating foods low in carbohydrates, which are essential for maintaining normal blood sugar levels. It has been shown to lower blood pressure, aid in weight loss & prevent heart disease and other chronic conditions. Additionally, the diet has been linked with a reduced risk of developing diabetes by lowering AGE (advanced glycation end products) levels, which are linked to various chronic diseases.
6. **Better Cholesterol Levels:** Following the Dash Diet can lead to higher HDL cholesterol levels compared to those following a typical diet. It has also been shown not only to lower LDL cholesterol and triglyceride levels, but also to raise DL cholesterol levels. Elevated triglyceride levels can ntribute to inflammation and plaque formation in arteries, increasing the risk of heart disease and stroke.
7. **Lower Risk of Chronic Diseases:** The Dash Diet is considered the optimal approach to reducing the risk of chronic diseases. By promoting healthy eating habits, this diet improves various aspects of overall health. It has been scientifically proven to lower blood pressure and cholesterol levels in healthy individuals, thereby preventing heart disease and diabetes. Additionally, the Dash Diet aids in improving body composition, which can further reduce the risk of cancer and other chronic diseases.
8. **Improved Sleep:** Unlike other diets, the Dash Diet has been shown to enhance sleep quality. Research indicates that individuals who adhere to the eating plan experience better sleep compared to those who don't. This improvement may be attributed to enhanced mood, increased serotonin levels, and reductions in inflammation and oxidative stress, which can interfere with quality sleep.

Food Guidelines

The DASH is a well-known diet that focuses on reducing high blood pressure. It emphasizes the consumption of nutrient-rich foods, including a balance of macronutrients: carbohydrates, proteins, and fats. Here's an explanation of the role of macronutrients and their correct balance in meals within the DASH diet:

1. **Carbohydrates:** These are a primary source of energy for the body. In the DASH diet, the emphasis is on consuming healthy, complex carbohydrates, such as whole grains, fruits, and vegetables. These provide essential vitamins, minerals, and fiber while having a lower impact on blood sugar levels compared to refined carbohydrates. The recommended balance of carbohydrates in the DASH diet is around 55-60% of total daily calories.
2. **Proteins:** Proteins are crucial for building and repairing tissues, supporting immune function, and producing enzymes and hormones. In the DASH diet, lean sources of protein, such as poultry, fish, legumes, and low-fat dairy products, are preferred over high-fat animal proteins. This helps reduce saturated and trans fats in the diet. The recommended balance of protein in the DASH diet is around 15-20% of total daily calories.
3. **Fats:** Fats provide energy, contribute in the absorption of fat-soluble vitamins and to hormone production. However, it's important to choose healthy fats and limit saturated and trans fats, as they

can increase the risk of cardiovascular disease. In the DASH diet, the focus is on consuming unsaturated fats, such as those found in olive oil, avocados, nuts, and seeds. The recommended balance of fats in the DASH diet is around 25-30% of total daily calories, with an emphasis on unsaturated fats.

Achieving a correct balance of macronutrients within the DASH diet involves planning meals that incorporate a variety of nutrient-dense foods. Here are some general tips:

1. To ensure you consume sufficient carbohydrates and fiber, make sure your plate is filled with vegetables, fruits, and whole grains.
2. Include lean sources of protein like poultry, fish, beans, and low-fat dairy products when planning your meals.
3. Moderately incorporate healthy fats such as olive oil, nuts, and seeds into your diet.
4. It is important to limit or avoid foods that are high in saturated and trans fats, including fatty meats, full-fat dairy products, and processed snacks.
5. Maintain a balanced calorie intake by being mindful of portion sizes.

Recommended Dash Diet Food List

1. **Vegetables:** Aim to have no more than forty-five percent of your meals to consist of vegetables; this is the minimum percentage you ought to shoot for. vegetables like broccoli, kale, collard greens, and leafy greens are examples. Asparagus, celery, and cucumbers, steaming spinach or green beans, and eggplant are all fantastic low-sodium food options. Eggplant is also a good choice.
2. **Fruits:** Fruits including apples, apricots, cherries, honeydew melon, grapefruit, oranges, tangerines, and pineapples. Avocado is beneficial due to the high levels of monounsaturated fat, protein, and fibre that it contains. When consumed in a responsible manner, bananas are another food that can be beneficial to your diet.
3. **Salad Greens:** including Romaine lettuce, Iceberg lettuce, Spinach, and Mixed Greens, etc. Combinations of different types of greens, like romaine lettuce and spinach, for example. Kale and spinach were blended in the dish. A delicious option to go with is a Greek salad. Broccoli, carrots, and bell peppers are just a few examples of veggies that taste delicious when grilled. In addition to being low in calories and rich in potassium and fibre, mushrooms are another healthy food option that should be considered.
4. **Soy and Pea Products:** tofu, edamame, tempeh, miso, shoyu (soy sauce), tempeh are high or good sources of protein.
5. **Legumes:** Soybeans, lentils, and beans are all examples of legumes, which provide phosphorus and fibre. They do this by interacting with cholesterols, which in turn raises the HDL (good) cholesterol level while simultaneously lowering the likelihood of type 2 diabetes. Grains are not only rich with complicated carbs but also an excellent source of protein.
6. **Vegetable Broth**: is a fine alternative provided that it does not include any extra MSG. Broths prepared from beans or vegetables ought to be drunk on a daily basis.
7. **Nuts:** are also a good choice. Almonds are one of the best choices because they are low in calories and contain monounsaturated fat and protein. They are high in calories, protein, fiber and monounsaturated fat.

8. **Whole Grain:** The inclusion of quinoa in a diet is recommended due to the grain's high levels of the nutrients fibre, calcium, and iron. Buckwheat and brown rice are both wonderful examples of foods that are rich in complex carbs. Consuming muesli and bread made with other whole grains on a daily basis is not uncommon.

9. **Drinks (water):** Hydration is essential to maintaining good health since it encourages people to ingest a greater number of vegetables and fruits, since they're the sole nutritious choices available to individuals who are not following a low-carb diet. Drinking water is crucial. On a low-carb diet, you should drink a lot of water as it helps you feel full and keeps you from eating too much. This will ensure that you do not go overboard with your food intake. Although it has no effect on weight, water can help suppress appetites and stop people from eating too much. People who drink water prior to meals tend to consume less food overall.

10. **Meat:** The Dash diet recommends that you continue to consume meat as part of your diet, but only in limited quantities each day. The quantity of meat that a person can consume is proportional to their age as well as their gender. It is suggested that women have one to one and a half oz. of lean muscle meat every day, whilst men ought to eat two to three oz. of lean muscle meat per day.

11. **Fish and Poultry:** You are allowed to have fish and poultry, but only in small quantities. One serving of fish is anywhere from three to four oz., while one serve of chicken is around the size of a deck of cards, which is approximately three ounces, or even less than that. Researches have indicated that eating fish twice per week is advantageous for heart health, particularly for younger women who are at risk for heart disease since they are more inclined to have high LDL cholesterol levels. This is particularly true for younger women who consume seafood. You can reduce the amount of saturated fat you eat by making seafood and poultry a regular part of your diet.

12. **Dairy:** The sole kinds of dairy products that are permitted on the Dash diet are fat-free or one percent milk or yoghurt, low-fat cheese, cottage cheese, part-skim mozzarella cheese, and soy products. You are additionally permitted to eat soy products. Products of the dairy industry that are fat-free or low-fat are your best option since, in comparison to full-fat dairy, they contain less saturated fat.

13. **Vegetable oil:** Approximately thirty calories and eight grams of total fat are found in one serving of vegetable oil. It is high in polyunsaturated fat, which is a healthy type of fat that has been demonstrated to lower the probability of developing cardiovascular disease. Olive oil, canola oil, soybean oil, and other forms of cooking oils are among the top goods. Other kinds of cooking oils also rank well.

Not Recommended for Dash Diet Food List

1. **Processed and High-Sodium Foods:** Packaged snacks, frozen meals, and canned soups are often packed with sodium. Consuming excessive sodium can contribute to elevated blood pressure, so it is advisable to minimize or avoid these items. Instead, prioritize fresh and whole foods, using herbs, spices, and other flavorings to enhance the taste of your dishes.

2. **Sugary Beverages and Sweets:** Sugar-sweetened beverages like soda, fruit juices, and energy drinks contain significant amounts of added sugars and empty calories. Similarly, desserts and sweets such as cakes, cookies, and candies can lead to weight gain and other health issues. Opt for water, unsweetened beverages, and naturally sweet treats like fresh fruits to satisfy your cravings.

3. **High-Fat Meats:** Fatty cuts of meat, including bacon, sausages, and processed meats like hot dogs and deli meats, tend to be high in saturated and trans fats. These fats can have adverse effects on heart health. Instead, turn to lean protein sources such as skinless poultry, fish, beans, and legumes.
4. **Full-Fat Dairy Products:** Full-fat dairy products like whole milk, cheese, and cream contain higher levels of saturated fats. These fats can contribute to increased cholesterol levels and a higher risk of heart disease. Opt for low-fat or fat-free dairy alternatives like skim milk, low-fat yogurt, and reduced-fat cheeses.
5. **Fried and Fast Foods:** Fried foods like French fries, fried chicken, and deep-fried snacks tend to be rich in unhealthy fats and calories. Fast food items such as burgers, pizza, and fried chicken are often processed, high in sodium, and generally unhealthy. It is best to limit or avoid these foods and instead prepare homemade meals using healthier cooking methods such as grilling, baking, or steaming.

Role of Salt

Salt, or sodium chloride, plays a vital role in the human body, including maintaining fluid balance, transmitting nerve impulses, and supporting muscle contractions. However, in the context of the DASH (Dietary Approaches to Stop Hypertension) diet, it is important to moderate salt intake to promote overall heart health. Here's an explanation of the role of salt in the body from a DASH diet perspective:

Salt, primarily composed of sodium, is an essential mineral that the body needs in small amounts to function properly. It helps maintain the balance of fluids within cells and throughout the body. Sodium plays a crucial role in nerve transmission, allowing electrical impulses to travel between cells, facilitating muscle contractions, including the heart, and supporting various biological processes.

However, excessive salt consumption has been linked to various health problems, particularly high blood pressure (hypertension). In the DASH diet, which aims to lower blood pressure, reducing sodium intake is a key principle. High sodium levels can cause fluid retention, leading to increased blood volume and subsequent elevated blood pressure. By lowering sodium intake, blood pressure can be better regulated, reducing the risk of cardiovascular issues.

The DASH diet recommends limiting sodium intake to no more than 2,300 milligrams (mg) per day, or even lower to 1,500 mg for individuals with hypertension, prehypertension, or those at higher risk of developing hypertension. This requires being mindful of the amount of sodium in foods consumed and making conscious choices to reduce salt intake.

To implement a low-sodium approach in the DASH diet, it is important to focus on consuming whole, unprocessed foods. Fresh fruits and vegetables, which are naturally low in sodium, can provide essential nutrients while adding flavor to meals. Whole grains, such as brown rice and quinoa, are another excellent choice as they are typically lower in sodium compared to processed grain products.

When cooking, it is advisable to minimize or eliminate the use of added salt. Instead, flavor dishes with herbs, spices, and other salt-free seasonings. Lemon juice, vinegar, and citrus zest can also enhance the taste of meals without the need for excessive sodium.

When selecting packaged foods, it becomes crucial to read labels carefully. Many processed foods, including snacks, sauces, condiments, and even seemingly healthy options, can be surprisingly high in sodium. Opting for low-sodium or sodium-free alternatives is a wiser choice within the DASH diet.

Recommended Daily Limits

Though the DASH diet primarily focuses on slashing sodium from the everyday diet, it also focuses on portion control and low-caloric intake. Portion control is essential for weight loss which is imperative to keeping blood pressure controlled. According to the NIH, a person should consume food as per the following serving sizes:

Grains: 6-8 Servings per Day

Grains are among the most consumed food groups, including rice, pasta, cereal, quinoa, bread, etc. Grains are a good source of complex carbs, fibers, some protein, minerals, and a few vitamins. Because of these benefits and the wide-ranging uses of grains in our diet, they are recommended for 6-8 servings per day. A single serving of grain means one slice of bread, one ounce of cereal, or half a cup of rice or pasta. Now multiply this serving size by 6 or 8 and divide the total amount into three-four meals of the day.

Vegetables: 4-5 Servings per Day

One cup of leafy vegetables and half a cup of other vegetables make one DASH diet serving. So, you can have two cups of vegetables and two cups of leafy greens per day on a dash diet. You can add these vegetables to the salads, pasta, and other savory delights.

Fruits: 4-5 Servings per Day

Half a cup of frozen or canned fruits and one cup of fresh fruit makes a single serving on a DASH diet. Since fruits are a major source of minerals, fibers, and vitamins, they must be consumed in 4-5 servings per day. Fruits are low on sodium and rich in fibers, so it is always healthy to consume them on the DASH diet.

Dairy: 2-3 Servings per Day

A single serving of dairy products on the DASH diet means one cup of low-fat yogurt, skimmed milk, or one and a half-ounce of part-skim cheese. So, you can consume 2-3 such servings in a day.

Nuts and Seeds: 4-5 Servings per Week

Legumes make a food group rich in carbs and plant-sourced proteins, including beans, lentils, split peas, etc. The legumes are paired with nuts and seeds to form one group, consumed in 4-5 servings per day on the DASH diet serving size formula.

Fats: 2-3 Servings per Day

Fats and oils contain three times the calories and energy than carbs; therefore, they must be consumed in a smaller amount in a day. For the Dash diet, 2-3 servings of fats and oil in any form is sufficient to meet the basic body needs. Try to add healthy unsaturated plant-based fats and oils to the diet to avoid bad cholesterols.

Sweets: 5 Servings or Fewer per Week

Sweets come last on this list, and they must be consumed in a very small amount on the dash diet. Five or fewer servings a week is sufficient to have on this diet. A single serving of sweet means half a cup of sorbet, one tablespoon of sugar, or one cup of sweet lemonade. So, you can have that single serving on alternate days of the week.

Sodium Recommendations

The goal is to reduce sodium intake to the point where it would stop interfering with the body's blood pressure levels. To achieve that, the DASH diet has two general recommendations:

- Standard: 2300mg or less of sodium per day.

- Low-Intake: 1500mg or less of sodium per day

Someone who is not suffering from hypertension can go with the 2300mg/day standard, while people with high blood pressure must consume 1500mg or less sodium in a day.

Shopping List

The DASH diet is all about loading up on fruits, vegetables, lean meats and fish, low-fat or fat-free dairy products, legumes, whole grains, seeds, and nuts. While those are strong foundations, it is just as important to make sure what you are eating is high in potassium, fiber, calcium, and magnesium in order to make sure that you are getting all of the possible health benefits from your food.

When it comes to fruits and vegetables, fresh is always best but we are not frowning upon frozen varieties as long as they have no added sugars, sauces, or anything. You want them to be as close to their natural state as possible, otherwise you would be cancelling out the health benefits from trying to cut back on sodium, saturated fats, and sugar. As far as dairy products go, just make sure they are either low-fat or fat-free alternatives. For whole-grains, just opt for whole-grain versions of your favorite pasta, bread, bagels, rice, and crackers. Finally, when it comes to seeds and nuts, make sure you are buying the unsalted, unflavored kinds.

Here are some of what you could be putting into your weekly grocery cart to ensure you are loading up on what is actually good for you:

Fruits:
- Apples
- Bananas
- Oranges
- Berries (strawberries, blueberries, raspberries)
- Grapes
- Melons (watermelon, cantaloupe)
- Citrus fruits (lemons, limes, grapefruits)

Vegetables:
- Leafy greens (spinach, kale, lettuce)
- Broccoli
- Carrots
- Tomatoes
- Cucumbers
- Bell peppers
- Onions
- Garlic
- Cauliflower
- Brussels sprouts

Whole Grains:
- Brown rice
- Quinoa
- Whole wheat bread
- Whole grain pasta
- Oats
- Barley
- Bulgur
- Whole grain cereals

Lean Proteins:
- Skinless chicken breasts
- Turkey breast
- Fish (salmon, tuna, trout)
- Shrimp
- Lean cuts of beef (loin, sirloin)
- Lean cuts of pork (loin, tenderloin)
- Eggs
- Tofu
- Beans and legumes (black beans, chickpeas, lentils)

Low-Fat Dairy or Dairy Alternatives:
- Skim milk
- Low-fat yogurt
- Low-fat cheese (cheddar, mozzarella)
- Greek yogurt
- Almond milk
- Soy milk
- Cottage cheese (low-fat or fat-free)

Nuts, Seeds, and Healthy Fats:
- Almonds
- Walnuts
- Pistachios
- Flaxseeds
- Chia seeds
- Avocados
- Olive oil
- Canola oil

Herbs, Spices, and Condiments:
- Basil
- Oregano
- Cumin
- Turmeric
- Cinnamon
- Black pepper
- Salt-free seasoning blends
- Vinegar (balsamic, apple cider, white)
- Mustard (Dijon, whole-grain)
- Low-sodium soy sauce
- Salsa (low-sodium)

Beverages:
- Water
- Herbal tea (unsweetened)
- Green tea
- Coffee (moderate consumption)

Snacks and Miscellaneous:
- Fresh or dried fruits (unsweetened)
- Raw vegetables for snacking
- Hummus (low-sodium)
- Whole grain crackers
- Air-popped popcorn (unsalted)
- Dark chocolate (70% cocoa or higher)

DASH Diet Success Stories

The DASH diet has garnered numerous success stories from individuals who have embraced this eating plan and experienced positive changes in their health. Here are a few inspiring stories:

Amanda's Story

Amanda's success story is a testament to the power of adopting a healthy eating plan, in this case, the DASH diet. At 60 years old, she decided to take control of her health after realizing the potential risks associated with being overweight and having high blood pressure.

The DASH diet, which stands for Dietary Approaches to Stop Hypertension, focuses on reducing fat intake while incorporating a variety of low-fat dairy products, fruits, and vegetables. Amanda embraced this eating plan and found it to be a game-changer for her weight loss journey and blood pressure management.

One of the key changes Amanda made was increasing her intake of fresh vegetables; she discovered her love for vegetables and began using them to fill her plate. While Amanda made a conscious effort to consume a balanced diet from all food groups, she found that vegetables became her go-to food and often served as her main course. She managed to incorporate other foods she enjoyed, such as meat and rice, but in smaller portions. Amanda mentions that she still allows herself to indulge in her beloved nachos occasionally, but she practices portion control to satisfy her cravings without derailing her progress.

What sets Amanda's success story apart is her realization that adopting a healthier way of eating doesn't mean completely giving up the foods she loves. By making smart choices, practicing moderation, and prioritizing nutrient-dense foods like vegetables, she was able to achieve her weight loss goals and significantly improve her blood pressure readings.

Amanda's enthusiasm and belief in the DASH diet are evident from her desire to become a spokesperson for the approach. Her success serves as an inspiration to others, demonstrating that with dedication and a balanced approach to eating, positive changes are possible at any age.

Ilary's Story

Ilary, a 45-year-old marketing executive from New York City, embarked on a transformative journey to improve her weight management and cardiovascular health. Frustrated with her sedentary lifestyle and unhealthy eating habits, Ilary decided it was time for a change.

Aware of the risks associated with excess weight and the impact it can have on heart health, Ilary sought a balanced approach that would address both her weight management goals and cardiovascular well-being.

After conducting extensive research and consulting with a nutritionist, Ilary devised a personalized plan that incorporated elements of the Mediterranean diet. This eating pattern emphasizes whole foods, lean proteins, fruits, vegetables, and healthy fats while limiting processed foods, added sugars, and saturated fats.

To kick-start her journey, Ilary began incorporating physical activity into her daily routine. Initially, she started with simple exercises like brisk walking and gradually progressed to more intense workouts such as cardio and strength training. Regular exercise not only helped Ilary shed excess pounds but also played a vital role in improving her cardiovascular fitness.

As Ilary embraced her new lifestyle, she discovered the joy of preparing wholesome meals. She focused on incorporating nutrient-dense foods into her diet, opting for colorful salads, grilled lean meats, and hearty vegetable-based soups. Portion control became an essential aspect of her eating habits, ensuring she consumed balanced meals without overindulging.

Over time, Ilary experienced remarkable progress. Her weight gradually decreased, and she felt more energized and confident. However, the most significant transformation came from within. Ilary's cardiovascular health showed significant improvements, with her blood pressure and cholesterol levels returning to healthy ranges.

Reflecting on her journey, Ilary emphasizes the importance of patience, consistency, and self-compassion. "It's not about deprivation or punishing yourself," she says. "It's about making sustainable changes that nourish your body and mind. Celebrate every small victory along the way, and remember that your health is a lifelong commitment."

Ilary's story serves as an inspiration for anyone seeking to manage their weight and improve cardiovascular health. By adopting a balanced approach, incorporating nutritious foods, staying active, and embracing self-care, it's possible to achieve lasting success and enjoy a vibrant, heart-healthy life.

Chapter 1. Breakfast Recipes

1. Breakfast Omelet

Preparation time: five mins
Cooking time: ten mins
Servings: two
Ingredients:

- 2 beaten eggs
- one stalk of green onion, sliced
- half teacup of mushrooms, sliced
- one red bell pepper, cubed
- one tsp of herb seasoning

Directions:

1. Put eggs in a dish.
2. Add the remaining components.
3. In a small baking pan.
4. Put in the basket, ten mins 350 deg. F in an oven.

Per serving: Calories: 48kcal; Carbs: 5g; Protein: 4g; Fat: 1g; Sodium: 23mg

2. Triple Berry Steel Cut Oats

Preparation time: five mins
Cooking time: four mins
Servings: 6
Ingredients:

- 2 cups of steel-cut oats
- three teacups of unsweetened almond milk
- three teacups water
- one tsp vanilla extract
- ⅓ cup of monk fruit sweetener
- ¼ teaspoon of salt
- one and half teacups of frozen berry blend with strawberries, blackberries, and raspberries

Directions:

1. Stir in the steel-cut oats, almond milk, water, vanilla, sweetener, and salt.
2. Add the frozen berries. Fix the lid and cook for four mins.
3. After fifteen mins, quick-release any leftover pressure until the float valve lowers, then open the lid.
4. Warm-up.

Per serving: Calories: 224kcal; Carbs: 42g; Protein: 7g; Fat: 3g; Sodium: 130mg

3. Breakfast Porridge

Preparation time: fifteen mins
Cooking time: zero mins
Servings: 1
Ingredients:

- six tbsps of organic cheese
- three tbsps of flax seed
- three tbsps of flax oil
- two tbsps of almond butter
- one tbsp of organic coconut meat
- one tbsp of raw honey
- quarter teacup water

Directions:

1. Inside a container, mix everything.
2. Mix thoroughly.
3. Serve in a chilled bowl.

Per serving: Calories: 180kcal; Carbs: 8g; Protein: 5g; Fat: 5g; Sodium: 100mg

4. Coconut Almond Granola

Preparation time: five mins
Cooking time: seven mins
Servings: 8
Ingredients:

- one and half teacups of rolled oats
- half teacup of unsweetened shredded coconut
- quarter teacup of monk fruit sweetener
- ⅛ teaspoon of salt
- three-quarter teacup almond butter
- quarter teacup of coconut oil

Directions:
1. Mix oats, coconut, sweetener, and salt inside a moderate container.
2. Mix in the almond butter and oil. Prepare cake pan with nonstick spray.
3. Add the oat mixture to the pot and cook for seven mins.
4. Cool thoroughly prior to serving.

Per serving: Calories: 155kcal; Carbs: 25g; Protein: 4gm; Fat: 8g; Sodium: 126mg

5. Breakfast Oatmeal

Preparation time: ten mins
Cooking time: fifteen mins
Servings: 6
Ingredients:

- 2/3 cup of coconut milk
- one egg white
- half teacup of gluten-free quick-cooking oats
- half tsp turmeric powder
- half tsp cinnamon
- quarter tsp ginger

Directions:
1. Heat non-dairy milk inside a saucepot across moderate flame.
2. Whisk in the egg white and continue whisking till uniform.
3. Add the other components and simmer for three mins.

Per serving: Calories: 184kcal; Carbs: 22g; Protein: 5g; Fat: 8g; Sodium: 138mg

6. Tomato Omelet

Preparation time: twenty mins
Cooking time: eight mins
Servings: one
Ingredients:

- two eggs
- half teacup basil, fresh
- half teacup of cherry tomatoes
- one tsp black pepper
- quarter teacup shredded cheese, any type
- half tsp salt
- two tbsps of olive oil

Directions:
1. Quarter the tomatoes. three mins in olive oil.
2. Set the tomatoes aside.
3. Whisk the eggs with salt & pepper inside a small container.
4. Pour the beaten egg solution into the pot then carefully work the edges beneath the omelet for three mins.
5. Add the basil, tomatoes, and cheese while the egg mixture is still runny.
6. Fold half the omelet across the other. Finished in two mins.

Per serving: Calories: 212kcal; Carbs: 26g; Protein: 22g; Fat: 11g; Sodium: 141mg

7. Breakfast Eggnog

Preparation time: five mins
Cooking time: zero mins
Servings: one
Ingredients:

- two eggs
- one teacup of rice milk, cold
- one tbsp of vanilla extract
- Sprint cinnamon
- Sprint nutmeg

Directions:

1. Blend the entire components inside a big cup or container till completely blended.
2. Serve with a tiny strainer into a serving glass.

Per serving: Calories: 126kcal; Carbs: 24g; Protein: 4g; Fat: 2g; Sodium: 7mg

8. Slow Cooker French Toast Casserole

Preparation time: fifteen mins
Cooking time: four mins
Servings: 9
Ingredients:

- two eggs
- 2 egg whites
- one and half almond milk
- two tbsps of honey
- ½ tsp cinnamon
- 1 tsp of vanilla extract
- 9 slices of bread

For filling:

- three teacups of apples (diced)
- two tbsps of raw honey
- one tbsp of lemon juice
- half tsp of cinnamon
- one-third teacup of pecans

Directions:

1. Mix the first six components.
2. Spray nonstick cooking spray on the slow cooker.
3. Set aside a small dish with all the filling components.
4. Coat the apple slices properly. Put three apple slices on the bottom of each triangle and some filing on top.
5. Stack the bread and filling in the same way.
6. Egg batter on the bread and filling layers.
7. Set the cooker for 2 1/two hrs on high or four hrs low.

Per serving: Calories: 252kcal; Carbs: 25g; Protein: 47.6g; Fat: 6g; Sodium: 155mg

9. Apple Cinnamon Steel Cut Oats

Preparation time: ten mins
Cooking time: four mins
Servings: 6
Ingredients:

- two teacups of steel-cut oats
- three teacups of unsweetened vanilla almond milk
- three teacups of water
- 3 small apples, cut into 1"-thick chunks
- two tsps of ground cinnamon
- quarter teacup of date syrup
- quarter tsp of salt

Directions:

1. Stir in the steel-cut oats, almond milk, water, apple pieces, cinnamon, date syrup, and salt.
2. Cook for ten mins.

Per serving: Calories: 112kcal; Carbs: 22g; Protein: 3g; Fat: 5g; Sodium: 146mg

10. Breakfast Casserole

Preparation time: ten mins
Cooking time: ten mins
Servings: 4
Ingredients:

- 1 lb. of hash browns
- 1 lb. of lean breakfast sausage, crumbled
- 1 yellow onion, sliced
- one red bell pepper, sliced
- 1 yellow bell pepper, sliced
- 1 green bell pepper, sliced
- Pepper

Directions:

1. Put hash browns, Sausage and vegetables for ten mins at 355 deg. F.
2. Add pepper and stir till it is completely cooked

Per serving: Calories: 40kcal; Carbs: 2g; Protein: 4g; Fat: 3g; Sodium: 21mg

11. Chia Breakfast Pudding

Preparation time: twenty mins
Cooking time: eight mins
Servings: one
Ingredients:

- 4 tablespoons of chia seeds
- one tbsp of almond butter
- three-quarter teacup coconut milk
- one tsp cinnamon
- one tsp vanilla
- three-quarter teacup cold coffee

Directions:

1. Pour the components into a refrigerator-safe container.
2. Cover and chill overnight.

Per serving: Calories: 220kcal; Carbs: 18g; Protein: 26g; Fat: 8g; Sodium: 161mg

12. Breakfast Stuffed Biscuits

Preparation time: thirty-five mins
Cooking time: thirty mins
Servings: 10
Ingredients:

- one tbsp of vegetable oil
- ¼ lb. of turkey sausage
- 2 beaten eggs
- Pepper
- 10 oz. frozen biscuits
- Cooking spray

Directions:

1. Cook sausage for five mins in hot oil in a medium skillet.
2. Set aside a bowl. Peppered eggs in a pan.
3. Pour eggs into the sausage dish.
4. Air fryer cookie dough Egg and sausage combination on top Seal the folds.
5. Oil spray for eight mins at 325 deg. F in an air fryer.
6. Cook for seven mins more.
7. Serve.

Per serving: Calories: 28kcal; Carbs: 8g; Protein: 6g; Fat: 5g; Sodium: 27mg

13. Ground Beef Breakfast Skillet

Preparation time: twenty mins
Cooking time: twenty mins
Servings: 4
Ingredients:

- one tbsp of olive oil
- one lb. of lean ground beef
- two tsps of minced garlic
- two teacups of chopped cauliflower
- one teacup of cubed carrots
- 1 zucchini, cubed
- Chopped white and green parts of 2 scallions

- Salt
- Ground black pepper
- two tbsps of chopped fresh parsley

Directions:
1. Heat the olive oil in a huge pan across moderate flame.
2. Add meat and garlic. Cook for eight mins or till done.
3. Be sure to mix in the veggies.
4. About ten mins till tender.
5. Add the scallions and sauté 1 minute.
6. Salt and pepper the mixture.
7. Garnish with parsley.

Per serving: Calories: 264kcal; Carbs: 45g; Protein: 8g; Fat: 4g; Sodium: 120mg

14. Pumpkin Quinoa Porridge

Preparation time: two mins
Cooking time: 1 minute
Servings: 4
Ingredients:

- three-quarter teacup dry quinoa
- two teacups water
- three-quarter teacup pumpkin purée
- quarter teacup monk fruit sweetener
- one and half tsps pumpkin pie spice
- one tsp pure vanilla extract
- quarter tsp salt

Directions:
1. Rinse the quinoa in a fine-mesh sieve 'til the water flows clear.
2. Quinoa, water, pumpkin purée, and salt to the inner saucepan.
3. Mix well and cook for 1 minute.
4. Allow quinoa to cool slightly prior to serving.

Per serving: Calories: 132kcal; Carbs: 17g; Protein: 3g; Fat: 5g; Sodium: 138mg

15. Gingerbread Oatmeal

Preparation time: ten mins
Cooking time: zero mins
Servings: one
Ingredients:

- one teacup water
- half teacup old-fashioned oats
- quarter teacup dried, unsweetened cranberries or cherries
- one tsp ground ginger
- half tsp ground cinnamon
- quarter tsp ground nutmeg
- one tbsp flaxseeds
- one tbsp molasses

Directions:
1. Combine the water, oats, ginger, cinnamon, and nutmeg in a small saucepan.
2. Bring to boil then lower the heat.
3. Simmer for five mins or till water is practically absorbed. Pour the flaxseeds.
4. Let it sit for five mins.
5. Before serving, spray with molasses.

Per serving: Calories: 316kcal; Carbs: 45g; Protein: 9g; Fat: 10g; Sodium: 400mg

16. Maple Oatmeal

Preparation time: five mins
Cooking time: twenty mins
Servings: 4
Ingredients:

- one tsp of maple flavoring
- one tsp Cinnamon
- three tbsps of Sunflower seeds
- half teacup chopped Pecans
- quarter teacup Coconut flakes, unsweetened
- half teacup chopped Walnuts

- half teacup milk, almond or coconut
- 4 tablespoons of Chia seeds

Directions:
1. Inside a mixing container, crush sunflower seeds, walnuts, and pecans.
2. Or put the nuts in a plastic bag, cover it in a towel, place it on a flat surface, and pound the cloth till the nuts shatter.
3. Pour the crushed nuts and the rest of the components into a big saucepan.
4. thirty mins on low heat with this combination. Stir often to prevent settling.
5. Garnish with fresh fruit or cinnamon if preferred.

Per serving: Calories: 182kcal; Carbs: 25g; Protein: 27g; Fat: 8g; Sodium: 181mg

17. Banana Chia Pudding

Preparation time: ten mins
Cooking time: zero mins
Servings: 3 glasses
Ingredients:

- two teacups of almond milk (unsweetened)
- half teacup of chia seeds
- 1 banana
- two tbsps of maple syrup
- half tsp of pure vanilla extract
- one tbsp of cacao powder

Mix-ins:

- two tbsps of cacao nibs
- two tbsps of chocolate chips
- 1 banana (sliced)

Directions:
1. Mix the chia seeds and bananas in a bowl. Mix them thoroughly.
2. Add vanilla and milk. Whisk till no lumps remain.
3. Prepare two re-sealable bags, one jar with half the chia seeds combination then pour with 1/2 chia seed combination with cacao powder and maple syrup.
4. Blend well into the second container and cover. Refrigerate for a few hours or overnight.
5. Divide the chia pudding across 3 glasses and top with the mix-ins. Serve.

Per serving: Calories: 112kcal; Carbs: 27g; Protein: 6g; Fat: 5g; Sodium: 96mg

18. Breakfast Tofu

Preparation time: forty mins
Cooking time: twenty mins
Servings: 4
Ingredients:

- two tsps of toasted sesame oil
- one tsp of rice vinegar
- two tbsps of soy sauce
- half tsp of onion powder
- one tsp of garlic powder
- 1 block of tofu
- one tbsp of potato starch

Directions:
1. All components except tofu and potato starch are in a bowl.
2. Blend well. Tofu in the bowl 30 min marinade Potato starch tofu.
3. Then add tofu. twenty mins at 370 deg. F, shaking midway.

Per serving: Calories: 226kcal; Carbs: 18g; Protein: 22g; Fat: 11g; Sodium: 133mg

19. At-Home Cappuccino

Preparation time: five mins
Cooking time: five mins
Servings: two
Ingredients:

- one teacup low-fat (1%) or fat-free milk
- 3 tbsp. ground espresso beans

Directions:
1. Heat the milk in a medium-hot saucepan till steaming. At the same time add cold water to the bottom of the coffee pot till the steam has evacuated.
2. Add the coffee beans to the basket and screw them on. Bring to a boiling point over high heat and cook till coffee stops splashing from the vertical flow under the lid. Eliminate from the heat.
3. Transfer the hot milk into a blender and mix till frothy.
4. Divide the coffee between two cups.
5. Pour in both cups the same amount of milk from the blender to cover the coffee, then pour in the remaining milk. Serve hot.

Per serving: Calories: 135kcal; Carbs: 17g; Protein: 10g; Fat: 2g; Sodium: 112mg

20. Blueberry Low-Sodium Pancakes

Preparation time: five mins
Cooking time: ten mins
Servings: 8
Ingredients:

- two teacups all-purpose flour
- 4 tbsp. brown sugar
- 2 tbsp. reduced sodium baking powder
- 1 tbsp. apple cider vinegar
- one tsp. vanilla extract
- one teacup oat milk

Directions:
1. Toss all the dry fixings (flour, brown sugar and baking powder) into a mixing container. Whisk till it's all blended.
2. In another mixing container or liquid measuring cup, add the wet fixings (oat milk, apple cider vinegar & vanilla), whisking till incorporated.
3. Combine all of the components till creamy. Wait while it rests (5 min.).
4. Pour the batter (1/2 cup) into a griddle or skillet using a medium-temperature setting.
5. Serve warm with honey or syrup.

Per serving: Calories: 177kcal; Carbs: 16g; Protein: 2g; Fat: 6g; Sodium: 113mg

21. Barley Porridge

Preparation time: five mins
Cooking time: twenty-five mins
Servings: 4
Ingredients:

- one teacup barley
- one teacup of wheat berries
- two teacups unsweetened almond milk
- two teacups of water
- one teacup toppings, such as hazelnuts, honey, berry, etc.

Directions:
1. Take a portable saucepan and put it on moderate-high flame. Add barley, almond milk, wheat berries, water, and bring to a boiling point.
2. Reduce the heat and wait for about twenty-five mins.
3. Divide into bowls then garnish with desired toppings.

Per serving: Calories: 295kcal; Carbs: 56g; Protein: 6g; Fat: 8g; Sodium: 110mg

22. Breakfast Frittata

Preparation time: fifteen mins
Cooking time: twenty mins
Servings: two
Ingredients:

- 1 onion, chopped
- two tbsps red bell pepper, chopped
- ¼ lb. breakfast turkey sausage, cooked and crumbled
- 3 eggs, beaten
- Pinch cayenne pepper

Directions:

1. Mix in a bowl. Pour into a baking dish.
2. Bake pan in air fryer basket, twenty mins in the air fryer.

Per serving: Calories: 200kcal; Carbs: 19g; Protein: 25g; Fat: 5g; Sodium: 151mg

23. Apples and Cinnamon Oatmeal

Preparation time: five mins
Cooking time: fifteen mins
Servings: two
Ingredients:

- one and half teacups unsweetened plain almond milk
- one teacup old-fashioned oats
- 1 large, unpeeled Granny Smith apple, cubed
- ¼ tsp. ground cinnamon
- 2 tbsp. toasted walnut pieces

Directions:

1. Bring the milk to warm across moderate flame and add the oatmeal and apple.
2. Whisk till almost all the liquid is absorbed, about four mins. Add the cinnamon.
3. Pour the oat mixture into two bowls and garnish with walnuts.

Per serving: Calories: 377kcal; Carbs: 73g; Protein: 13g; Fat: 16g; Sodium: 77mg

24. Apple Oats

Preparation time: ten mins
Cooking time: seven mins
Servings: two
Ingredients:

- 2 apples, cored, peeled, and cubed
- one teacup gluten-free oats
- one and half teacups of water
- one and half teacups of almond milk
- 2 tbsp. swerve
- 2 tbsp. almond butter
- ½ tsp. cinnamon powder
- 1 tbsp flax seed, ground
- Cooking spray

Directions:

1. With cooking spray, grease a slow cooker and toss the oat with the water and other components inside. Stir a little and simmer for seven mins.
2. Divide into bowls and serve for breakfast.

Per serving: Calories: 140kcal; Carbs: 28g; Protein: 5g; Fat: 4g; Sodium: 44mg

25. Breakfast Rice Porridge

Preparation time: 10minutes
Cooking time: twenty-five mins
Servings: two
Ingredients:

- 2 dates, chopped
- 1 oz. of protein powder, unflavored
- one and half teacups of almond milk, unsweetened
- half teacup of short grain brown rice
- 1 medium-sized banana, sliced
- one tbsp of tahini

- 1 apple, chopped
- one tsp of sesame seeds, toasted

Directions:
1. Put rice, almond milk, and protein powder in a large pot.
2. Cook for twenty to twenty-five mins or 'til the rice is done. Stir often.
3. Serve the rice porridge with the fruits and dates.
4. Garnish with sesame seeds and tahini.

Per serving: Calories: 140kcal; Carbs: 28g; Protein: 8g; Fat: 2g; Sodium: 120mg

Chapter 2. Recipes for Lunches

26. Pork with Scallions and Peanuts
Preparation time: ten mins
Cooking time: 16 minutes
Servings: 4
Ingredients:

- two tbsps lime juice
- two tbsps coconut amino
- one and half tbsps brown sugar
- 5 garlic cloves, minced
- three tbsps olive oil
- Black pepper to the taste
- 1 yellow onion, cut into wedges
- 1/2-pound pork tenderloin, cubed
- three tbsps peanuts, chopped
- 2 scallions, chopped

Directions:
1. Mix lime juice with amino and sugar in a bowl and stir very well.
2. Mix garlic with one and half tsps oil and some black pepper in another bowl and stir.
3. Add one onion and mix it.
4. Add the garlic mix, return the pork, add the amino mix, toss, cook for 6 minutes, divide between plates, sprinkle scallions and peanuts on top and serve.

Per serving: Calories: 273kcal; Carbs: 12g; Protein: 18g; Fat: 4g; Sodium: 162mg

27. Creamy Smoky Pork Chops
Preparation time: ten mins
Cooking time: twenty mins
Servings: 4
Ingredients:

- two tbsps olive oil
- 4 pork chops
- one tbsp chili powder
- Black pepper to the taste
- one tsp sweet paprika
- 1 garlic clove, minced
- one teacup coconut milk
- one tsp liquid smoke
- 1/4 cup cilantro (chopped)
- Juice of 1 lemon

Directions:
1. Mix pork chops with pepper, chili powder, paprika, and garlic in a bowl and rub well.
2. Heat a pan with the oil over moderate-high flame, add pork chops then cook for five mins on each side.
3. Inside a mixer, mix coconut milk with liquid smoke, lemon juice and cilantro, blend well, pour across the chops, cook for ten mins more, divide everything between plates and serve.

Per serving: Calories: 240kcal; Carbs: 10g; Protein: 22g; Fat: 8g; Sodium: 132mg

28. Southwestern Chicken and Pasta
Preparation time: ten mins
Cooking time: twenty mins
Servings: two
Ingredients:

- one teacup uncooked whole-wheat rigatoni
- 2 chicken breasts, cut into cubes
- quarter teacup of salsa
- one and half teacups of canned unsalted tomato sauce
- one-eighth tsp garlic powder

- one tsp cumin
- half tsp chili powder
- half teacup canned black beans, drained
- half teacup fresh corn
- quarter teacup Monterey jack and Colby cheese, shredded

Directions:
1. Fill a pot with water up to ¾ full and boil it. Add pasta to cook till it is al dente, then drain the pasta while rinsing under cold water. Preheat a skillet with cooking oil, then cook the chicken for ten mins till golden from both sides.
2. Add tomato sauce, salsa, cumin, garlic powder, black beans, corn, and chili powder. Cook the mixture while stirring, then toss in the pasta. Serve with two tablespoons of cheese on top. Enjoy.

Per serving: Calories: 245kcal; Carbs: 19.3g; Protein: 33.3g; Fat: 16.3g; Sodium: 515mg

29. Spiced Winter Pork Roast

Preparation time: fifteen mins
Cooking time: twenty mins
Servings: 6
Ingredients:

- 2 ½ pounds pork roast
- Black pepper to the taste
- one tsp chili powder
- half tsp onion powder
- quarter tsp cumin, ground
- one tsp cocoa powder

Directions:
1. Combine the roast with black pepper, chili powder, onion powder, cumin and cocoa, rub, cover the pan, place into oven and cook it for twenty mins.
2. Slice, divide between plates and serve with a side salad.

Per serving: Calories: 288kcal; Carbs: 12g; Protein: 23g; Fat: 5g; Sodium: 82mg

30. Pork Chops And Apples

Preparation time: ten mins
Cooking time: 1 hour
Servings: 4
Ingredients:

- one and half teacups chicken stock
- Black pepper to the taste
- 4 pork chops
- 1 yellow onion, chopped
- one tbsp olive oil
- 2 garlic cloves, minced
- 3 apples, cored and sliced
- one tbsp thyme, chopped

Directions:
1. Heat a pan with the oil over moderate-high flame, add pork chops, season with black pepper and cook for five mins.
2. Add onion, garlic, apples, thyme and stock, toss, introduce in the oven and bake at 350 deg. F for fifty mins. Divide everything between plates and serve.

Per serving: Calories: 332kcal; Carbs: 50g; Protein: 7.4g; Fat: 13.7g; Sodium: 226mg

31. Shrimp with Garlic and Mushrooms

Preparation time: fifteen mins
Cooking time: twenty mins
Servings: 4 people
Ingredients:

- one teacup extra-virgin olive oil
- quarter tsp salt
- one lb. peeled and deveined fresh shrimp
- 8 large garlic cloves, thinly sliced

- quarter teacup chopped fresh flat-leaf Italian parsley
- half tsp red pepper flakes
- 4 ounces sliced mushrooms
- Zucchini noodles or riced cauliflower, for serving

Directions:
1. Clean the shrimp by rinsing them and patting them dry. Put inside a blending container with a tweak of salt. Heat the olive oil over medium-low heat in a huge rimmed, thick skillet.
2. Bring to the boil for four - five mins, or till extremely fragrant, lowering the fire if the garlic begins to burn.
3. Pour the mixture and cook for another five mins, or till they are softened. Add the prawns and red pepper seasoning and cook for yet another 4 - five mins, or till the shrimp becomes pink.
4. Served with mid-engine cauliflower.

Per serving: Calories: 353kcal; Carbs: 4g; Protein: 24g; Fat: 26g; Sodium: 865mg

32. Thai Curry with Prawns

Preparation time: twenty mins
Cooking time: thirty mins
Servings: two
Ingredients:

- one tbsp coconut oil
- one red pepper cut into roughly 1" chunks
- 4 spring onions thickly sliced
- four tsps root ginger, peeled and finely grated
- 3 tablespoon Thai red curry paste
- ½ can use coconut milk of about one and three-quarter teacups
- three-quarter teacup mange tout or sugar snap peas, halved
- one red chili, finely sliced
- one and two-third teacups of cooked prawns

Directions:
1. Take a big nonstick frying pan, heat the oil across moderate-high flame and stir-fry the pepper for two mins.
2. Cook for another min, constantly stirring, once including the spring onions, ginger, and curry paste.
3. Fill the pan midway with coconut milk and raise to a medium simmer. Add the mange tout or sugar snap peas and the chili if using.
4. Return to low heat then cook for additional two mins, mixing irregularly. Heat for one–two mins or till the prawns are warmed.
5. If the sauce becomes thick, too, add a drop of water. Serve with cauliflower rice that has just been cooked.

Per serving: Calories: 374kcal; Carbs: 13.5g; Protein: 9g; Fat: 21g; Sodium: 352mg

33. Ginger And Chili Baked Fish

Preparation time: thirty mins
Cooking time: forty mins
Servings: one
Ingredients:

- two tsps olive oil
- 6 ounces thick white fish fillet,
- 1 garlic clove, peeled and thinly sliced
- three tsps of stem ginger
- 1 spring onion
- one red bird's eye chili,
- ½ small lime
- Handful fresh coriander leaves
- Pepper as required
- quarter salt

Directions:
1. Warm up the oven to 400 deg F. Spray the oil over a rectangle of kitchen foil on a baking tray. Put the fish on half of the foil, skin side down, with sufficient foil to cover it. Garlic, ginger, spring onion, and chili are sprinkled across the fish, and lime juice is squeezed over it.
2. Toss the fish with salt and black pepper prior to folding the foil over it and rolling up the edges to seal it within. Because steam is required to cook the fish, make sure the package isn't too tight. Oven preheated to 350 deg F and bake the fish for approximately twenty mins, or till a fork pierces the fish and it flakes into big pieces.
3. Using a fish slice carefully open the foil bundle and lift the fish onto a warming platter. Serve the fish with the cooking fluids, lots of fresh coriander, and lime wedges on the side.

Per serving: Calories: 233kcal; Carbs: 7g; Protein: 31g; Fat: 11g; Sodium: 346mg

34. Beef Stroganoff

Preparation time: thirty-five mins
Cooking time: fifty mins
Servings: two
Ingredients:

- 9 ounces sirloin steak
- two tbsps olive oil
- one average onion, skinned and finely cut
- 5 ounces button chestnut mushrooms, sliced
- one tsp paprika (not smoked)
- 2/3 cup beef stock (made with ½ beef stock cube)
- two tsps cornflour
- two tbsps full-Protein: crème Fraiche
- Chopped fresh parsley to serve
- quarter salt
- Pepper as required

Directions:
1. Eliminate any extra Protein: from the steak and cut it into long, thin strips that are no more than ½" broad on a slight diagonal. Season with salt and ground black pepper.
2. Use a nonstick frying pot, and heat one tbsp of the oil across moderate-high flame. Cook for two–three mins, or till the steak is browned but not cooked through. Return the pan to heat and remove the steak to a platter.
3. Cook for four–five mins, or till the onions are softened and mildly browned, using the remaining oil in the pan is onion and mushrooms.
4. Cook for a few more seconds once including the paprika.
5. Bring the broth to a low fire in the pan. Cook, frequently stirring, for two mins.
6. Mix the cornflour and one tbsp of fresh water in a small dish, then stir into the pan. Put the steak in the pan with the crème Fraiche. Warm the meat in the sauce for one–two mins, stirring frequently then adding a splash of water if necessary. To serve, garnish with chopped fresh parsley.

Per serving: Calories: 394kcal; Carbs: 33g; Protein: 22g; Fat: 11g; Sodium: 56mg

35. Chicken Veronique

Preparation time: ten mins
Cooking time: twenty-seven mins
Servings: 5
Ingredients:

- one tbsp flour
- one bay leaf

- quarter tsp pepper
- half teacup water
- one lb. chicken breast meat
- six tbsps unsalted margarine
- 1/4 cup white wine
- one tsp parsley
- quarter tsp pepper
- two tbsps orange marmalade
- one teacup halved white grapes

Directions:
1. Combine flour and quarter tsp pepper inside a blending container. Dust the chicken with a light coating of flour. In a large pot, cook the chicken in margarine till golden brown on both ends.
2. Except for the grapes, blend the remaining components. Cover then cook for twenty-five mins or till the vegetables are soft. Put the chicken on a serving plate.
3. Cook for two mins, stirring regularly, once including the grapes to the gravy. Pour the sauce across the chicken.

Per serving: Calories: 274kcal; Carbs: 13g; Protein: 22g; Fat: 13g; Sodium: 86mg

36. Chicken Chili

Preparation time: fifteen mins
Cooking time: twenty mins
Servings: 10
Ingredients:

- four tbsps extra-virgin olive oil
- 6 cloves garlic, crushed
- 2 medium green bell peppers, severed
- two big onions, severed
- four teacups cubed sweet potatoes
- four tsps ground cumin
- four tbsps chili powder
- two tsps dried oregano
- 2 cans (15 oz each) of low-sodium cannellini beans, rinsed
- two teacups frozen corn
- half tsps salt
- four teacups chicken stock
- four teacups cooked, cubed chicken
- half tsp pepper or as required

To serve:
- Sour cream
- Chopped cilantro
- Avocado, skinned, pitted, severed

Directions:
1. Whisk oil into a big soup pot and warm across the flame. Once the oil is heated, include garlic & onion then cook for a few mins.
2. Stir in sweet potatoes and bell pepper and cook till vegetables are mildly cooked. Include spices and oregano and stir for a few seconds till you get a nice aroma.
3. Stir in beans and broth. Slow down the heat, cover the pot partially and cook for around twenty mins once it starts to boil. Include corn and cook for a few mins. Stir in chicken and heat thoroughly.
4. Turn off the heat. Include salt and pepper and stir. Ladle into bowls.
5. Serve with suggested toppings.

Per serving: Calories: 365kcal; Carbs: 47g; Protein: 15g; Fat: 13g; Sodium: 351mg

37. Mediterranean Fish Bake

Preparation time: twenty mins
Cooking time: forty-five mins
Servings: two
Ingredients:

- one average red onion cut into 12 parts
- one red pepper cut into roughly 1" chunks

- 1 courgette halved lengthways and cut into roughly 1" chunks
- 2 medium tomatoes, quartered
- 1½ tablespoon olive oil
- 4 oz. of sea bass or sea bream fillets
- three tbsps pitted black olives (preferably Kalamata), drained
- Juice ½ large lemon, plus extra wedges to serve
- quarter salt and pepper as required

Directions:
1. Warm up the oven to 400 deg F. Scatter the onion, pepper, courgette and tomato quarters on a large baking tray. Toss everything together with one tbsp of oil sprayed on top. Roast for twenty mins, seasoning with sea salt & freshly ground black pepper.
2. Retrieve the dish from the oven and season the fish with pepper prior to placing it skin-side downwards amongst some vegetables. Sprinkle the olives on top after squeezing the lemon zest across the top.
3. Return the dish to the oven there for another approximately ten mins till either the vegetables are supple or the salmon is cooked through. Serve the fish and veggies on two hot plates with the remaining oil sprayed on top and lemon wedges on the side.

Per serving: Calories: 274kcal; Carbs: 22g; Protein: 11g; Fat: 26g; Sodium: 146mg

38. Baked Salmon

Preparation time: ten mins
Cooking time: 1 hour fifty mins
Servings: four
Ingredients:

- four oz. salmon fillets
- two pieces garlic
- three tbsps olive oil
- one tsp basil leave
- quarter tsp black pepper
- half tbsp lemon juice
- half tbsp parsley (severed)
- quarter salt (optional)

Directions:
1. Prepare the marinade inside a moderate container by combining garlic, olive oil, basil leaves, salt, pepper, lemon juice, and parsley.
2. Put the salmon fillets with the marinade in a medium glass baking dish. Marinate for one hr in the refrigerator, rotating periodically. Warm up the oven to 375 deg. F.
3. Fill the aluminum foil with fillets, top with marinade, and seal. Put the sealed salmon in the dish and bake for a minimum of thirty-five mins or till fork-tender.

Per serving: Calories: 244kcal; Carbs: 1g; Protein: 21g; Fat: 2g; Sodium: 56mg

39. Healthy, Juicy Salmon Dish

Preparation time: five mins
Cooking time: thirteen mins
Servings: one
Ingredients:

- quarter teacup water
- Few sprigs of parsley, basil, and tarragon
- 0.5 pounds of salmon (skin on)
- one tsp ghee
- one tsp salt
- two tbsps + two tsps of pepper
- quarter lemon (finely cut)
- 0.5 whole carrot (julienned)

Directions:
1. Include water and herbs to your pot and set it to Sauté mode. Put the salmon on a steamer rack inside your pot. Season the salmon with salt & pepper then spray with ghee.
2. Put the slices of lemon on top. Cook for almost three mins on HIGH pressure with the cover locked on the pot. Allow ten mins for the pressure to dissipate naturally.
3. Put it on a serving plate and serve. Include carrots, parsley, basil, and tarragon to your pot in Sauté mode.
4. Cook for one-two mins prior to serving the salmon on a dish. Serve.

Per serving: Calories: 464kcal; Carbs: 3gm; Protein: 34g; Fat: 34g; Sodium: 466mg

40. Sesame Salmon With Broccoli And Tomatoes

Preparation time: thirty mins
Cooking time: twenty-five mins
Servings: two
Ingredients:

- two tsps rapeseed oil
- two pieces of salmon fillets
- 6 spring onions
- 12 tomatoes
- 7 oz. broccoli, trimmed
- one tbsp soya sauce
- one tsp Sesame oil
- half tsp crushed dried chili flakes
- one tsp sesame seeds

Directions:
1. Warm up the oven to 400 deg F. Spray the oil over a baking tray. Put the salmon fillets down in the tray, along with the spring onions and tomatoes, and season generously with ground black pepper.
2. Heated the oven to 350 deg F and bake for eight mins. In the meantime, fill a pan midway with water and raise it to a boil. Return the pot to a boil with the broccoli.
3. Drain after four mins of cooking. Put the broccoli on the baking tray after removing it from the oven.
4. Soya sauce and sesame oil should be sprayed across the fish. Revert the salmon to the oven for the next 3 to four mins, or till just done, then sprinkle with the chili powder and sesame seeds.
5. Split it up between two heated plates to serve.

Per serving: Calories: 224kcal; Carbs: 20gm; Protein: 17g; Fat: 21g; Sodium: 196mg

41. Mediterranean Pork

Preparation time: ten mins
Cooking time: thirty-five mins
Servings: two
Ingredients:

- two pork chops (bone-in)
- half tsp salt pepper as required
- one and half garlic cloves (skinned and crushed)
- half tsp dried rosemary

Directions:
1. Warm up the oven to 425 deg. F. Sprinkle on the pork chops with salt and pepper. Include rosemary and garlic to them in a roasting pan.
2. Cook for ten mins in the oven and then diminish the heat to 350 F then roast for another twenty-five mins.
3. Pork chops should be sliced and served on plates. Spray the pan liquid all across the place. Serve.

Per serving: Calories: 335kcal; Carbs: 1.52g; Protein: 40.48g; Fat: 17.42g; Sodium: 126mg

42. Tuna and Potato Bake

Preparation time: ten mins
Cooking time: forty mins
Servings: two
Ingredients:

- one lb. boiled potatoes
- one average onion
- 20 ounces tin of tuna (drained)
- ½ lemon juice
- 2 tweaks nutmeg
- Black pepper as required
- 4 eggs (beaten)
- Butter/margarine as required

Directions:

1. Cook the onion for ten mins at a low temperature. Combine the onion and potato inside a blending container. Blend the pepper, lemon juice, nutmeg, and beaten eggs inside a blending container.
2. Toss the tuna with the potato mixture and flake it up. Brush the top of the mixture with melted butter or margarine and place it in an ovenproof dish that has been properly buttered.
3. Warm up the oven to about 400 deg F (Gas Mark 6) then bake for thirty mins till the top is well browned.

Per serving: Calories: 521kcal; Carbs: 70g; Protein: 76g; Fat: 6g; Sodium: 146mg

43. Mussels with Tomatoes & Chili

Preparation time: fifteen mins
Cooking time: twelve mins
Servings: 4
Ingredients:

- two ripe tomatoes
- two tbsps olive oil
- one tsp tomato paste
- 1 garlic clove (severed)
- 1 shallot (severed)
- 1 severed red or green chili
- A small glass of dry white wine
- 2 lbs. mussels, cleaned
- Basil leaves
- quarter salt and pepper as required

Directions:

1. Include tomatoes to boiling water for three mins, then drain. Peel the tomatoes and chop the flesh. Include oil to an iron griddle and heat to sauté shallots and garlic for three mins.
2. Stir in wine and tomatoes, chili, salt & pepper, and tomato paste. Cook for two mins, then include mussels. Garnish with basil leaves and serve warm.

Per serving: Calories: 270kcal; Carbs: 12g; Protein: 23g; Fat: 15.2gm; Sodium: 36mg

44. Currant Pork Chops

Preparation time: ten mins
Cooking time: twenty mins
Servings: 6
Ingredients:

- two tbsps Dijon mustard
- 6 pork loin chops, center cut
- two tsps olive oil
- one-third teacup wine vinegar
- quarter teacup black currant jam
- 6 orange slices
- one-eighth tsp black pepper

Directions:

1. Start by mixing your mustard and jam in a bowl.
2. Get out a nonstick griddle, and oil it with olive oil prior to placing it across moderate

flame. Cook your chops for five mins per side, and then top with a tablespoon of the jam mixture. Cover, and allow it to cook for two mins. Transfer them to a serving plate.

3. Pour your wine vinegar in the same griddle, and scape the bits up to deglaze the pan, mixing well. Spray this over your pork chops.
4. Garnish with pepper and orange slices prior to serving warm.

Per serving: Calories: 265kcal; Carbs: 11g; Protein: 25g; Fat: 6g; Sodium: 12mg

45. Chicken Divan

Preparation time: fifteen mins
Cooking time: thirty mins
Servings: two
Ingredients:

- half-pound cooked chicken, boneless, skinless, diced in bite-size pieces
- one teacup broccoli, cooked, diced into bite-size parts
- one teacup extra sharp cheddar cheese, grated
- 1 can mushroom soup
- half teacup of water
- one teacup croutons

Directions:

1. Warm the oven to 350 deg. F.
2. Inside a big saucepan, bring the soup and water to a simmer. Next, stir in the chicken, broccoli, and cheese.
3. Completely mix the components. Pour onto a baking dish that has been buttered.
4. The croutons should be placed on top of the solution.
5. Bake for approximately thirty mins, or till the casserole is bubbling and the croutons have reached the desired color.

Per serving: Calories: 380kcal; Carbs: 10g; Protein: 25g; Fat: 22g; Sodium: 397mg

46. Crunchy Fish Bites

Preparation time: twenty-five mins
Cooking time: thirty mins
Servings: two
Ingredients:

- one average egg
- three tbsps quick-cook polenta (fine cornmeal)
- four tsps of ground almonds
- 10 oz. thick skinless white fish fillet (like cod, haddock or Pollock), cut into roughly 1 ½" chunks
- two tbsps olive or rapeseed oil
- Lemon wedges, to serve
- half tsp

Directions:

1. Use a small container, whisk the egg and season with salt and pepper. Inside a separate container, blend the polenta and almonds. Season with black pepper and sea salt.
2. Turn the pieces of fish in the beaten egg one at a time till thoroughly coated, then in the polenta mixture.
3. Put on a platter and set away. Put a big nonstick frying pot across moderate flame and pour the oil.
4. Fry the fish bites for five–seven mins, depending on thickness, till cooked through, golden brown, and crisp on all sides, flipping occasionally. Lemon is also served on the side for squeezing.

Per serving: Calories: 384kcal; Carbs: 15g; Protein: 33g; Fat: 0g; Sodium: 99mg

47. Mediterranean Beef Dish

Preparation time: ten mins
Cooking time: fifteen mins
Servings: 3
Ingredients:

- one-third lb. beef, ground
- half teacup zucchinis, severed
- quarter teacup yellow onion, severed
- quarter tsp salt and black pepper as required
- 3 ounces canned roasted tomatoes and garlic
- quarter teacup of water
- quarter teacup cheddar cheese, shredded
- half teacup white rice

Directions:

1. Warm a pot across moderate-high flame, include beef, onion, salt, pepper, and zucchini, stir and cook for seven mins.
2. Include water, tomatoes, and garlic, stir and raise to a boil. Include rice, more salt, and pepper, stir, cover, take off the heat and leave aside for seven mins.
3. Divide between plates and serve with cheddar cheese on top.

Per serving: Calories: 278kcal; Carbs: 28g; Protein: 27g; Fat: 7g; Sodium: 72mg

48. Smoked Salmon Crudités

Preparation time: ten mins
Cooking time: fifteen mins
Servings: four
Ingredients:

- six oz. smoked wild salmon
- 1 tbsp. severed scallions (green parts only)
- 2 tbsp. roasted garlic aioli
- 2 tsp. severed capers
- 1 tbsp. Dijon mustard
- 4 endive spears or hearts of romaine
- half English cucumber (cut into quarter inch dense rounds)
- ½ tsp. dried dill

Directions:

1. Cut the smoked salmon into small parts then put inside a small container. Mix in the scallions, aioli, capers, Dijon and dill till thoroughly blended.
2. Serve chilled with a teaspoon of smoked salmon mixture on top of endive spears and cucumber rounds.

Per serving: Calories: 95kcal; Carbs: 1g; Protein: 6g; Fat: 6g; Sodium: 38mg

49. Balsamic-Roasted Chicken Breasts

Preparation time: thirty mins
Cooking time: forty mins
Servings: two
Ingredients:

- quarter teacup balsamic vinegar
- one tbsp olive oil
- two tsps dried oregano
- four garlic pieces, crushed
- one-eighth tsp salt
- half tsp freshly ground black pepper
- 2 (four oz.) boneless, skinless, chicken breast halves
- Cooking spray

Directions:

1. Include olive oil, vinegar, oregano, garlic, salt, and pepper inside a small container. Mix to blend.
2. Put the chicken in a plastic bag that can be resealed. Fill the bag with the vinegar mixture and the chicken, close it, and marinate the chicken. Refrigerate for thirty mins prior to serving.

3. Disperse a baking dish with cooking spray.
4. Pour the marinade across the chicken, put the chicken in a prepared baking dish cover and bake r till an instant-read thermometer registers 165 deg. F.
5. Wait for five mins, then serve with your favorite vegetables.

Per serving: Calories: 226kcal; Carbs: 6g; Protein: 25g; Fat: 11g; Sodium: 129mg

50. Sesame Chicken Veggie Wraps

Preparation time: ten mins
Cooking time: five – ten mins
Servings: four
Ingredients:
For dressing:

- one tbsp orange juice
- half tsp sesame oil
- one tbsp olive oil
- A tweak pepper
- quarter tsp ground ginger
- quarter tsp salt

For wraps:

- 4 whole-wheat tortillas (8 inches each)
- half teacup frozen shelled edamame
- one teacup fresh baby spinach
- half teacup severed, fresh sugar snap peas
- quarter teacup finely cut sweet red pepper
- half teacup finely cut cucumber
- quarter teacup shredded carrots
- half teacup cooked, severed chicken breast

Directions:
1. Follow the directions on the package then cook the edamame. Drain in a colander then wash under cold running water.
2. Whisk together orange juice, sesame oil, olive oil, pepper, ginger, and salt inside a container.
3. Put drained edamame, chicken, spinach, sugar snap peas, red pepper, cucumber, and carrots inside a container and whisk thoroughly.
4. Warm the tortillas according to the package recommendations. Disperse the vegetable mixture on the tortillas. Wrap like a burrito and serve.

Per serving: Calories: 214kcal; Carbs: 28g; Protein: 12g; Fat: 7g; Sodium: 229mg

Chapter 3. Recipes for Dinners

51. Chicken Tomato and Green Beans

Preparation time: fifteen mins
Cooking time: twenty-five mins
Servings: two
Ingredients:

- 6 oz. low-sodium canned tomato paste
- two tbsps olive oil
- quarter tsp black pepper
- two lbs. trimmed green beans
- two tbsps severed parsley
- one and half lbs. boneless, skinless, and cubed chicken breasts
- 25 oz. no-salt-included canned tomato sauce

Directions:
1. Include chicken, stir, cover, cook within five mins on both sides and transfer it to a container and warm the oil. Include and heat the green beans in the same griddle with the remaining oil across moderate flame, stir and cook for ten mins.
2. Return the chicken to the pan, include black pepper, tomato sauce, tomato paste, and parsley, stir, cover, cook for ten more mins, split between plates, and serve. Enjoy!

Per serving: Calories: 190kcal; Carbs: 14g; Protein: 9gm; Fat: 4g; Sodium: 168mg

52. Pork Strips and Rice

Preparation time: ten mins
Cooking time: twenty-five mins
Servings: one
Ingredients:

- half lb. pork loin, cut into strips
- quarter tsp salt and pepper as required
- one tbsp olive oil
- one carrot, severed
- one red bell pepper, severed
- 2 garlic pieces, crushed
- half teacup veggie stock
- quarter teacup basmati rice
- quarter teacup garbanzo beans
- 2 black olives, pitted and sliced
- one tbsp parsley, severed

Directions:
1. Warm a pot with the oil across moderate-high flame.
2. Include the pork fillets, stir, cook for five mins and transfer them to a plate.
3. Include the carrots, bell pepper, and garlic, stir and cook for five more mins.
4. Include the rice, the stock, beans, and the olives, stir, cook for fourteen mins, split between plates, sprinkle the parsley across the top and serve.

Per serving: Calories: 220kcal; Carbs: 7gm; Protein: 11g; Fat: 12g; Sodium: 102mg

53. Fish with Peppers

Preparation time: ten mins
Cooking time: twenty mins
Servings: 5
Ingredients:

- one and half lbs. fish fillets
- one tsp garlic powder
- half teacup low-sodium chicken broth
- quarter teacup no-salt-included tomato sauce
- one tsp capers

- two tbsps oil
- half tsp lemon pepper
- half average green pepper (cut into rings)
- half average red pepper (cut into rings)

Directions:
1. Cut the fish into 4-inch chunks. Inside a big pot, cook the salmon in oil for five mins across moderate flame, flipping often.
2. Blend the broth, tomato sauce, and capers in a large mixing bowl. Diminish the heat to low, cover, then cook for ten mins.
3. Cook for another five mins, or 'til the fish flakes simply with a fork and soft peppers.

Per serving: Calories: 205kcal; Carbs: 8g; Protein: 23g; Fat: 11g; Sodium: 136mg

54. Taco-Seasoned Roast Beef Wraps

Preparation time: ten mins
Cooking time: zero mins
Servings: two
Ingredients:

- two tbsps low-fat cream cheese
- 2 (10-inch) flour tortillas
- 4 ounces low-sodium roast beef
- half teacup fresh spinach
- one tsp Taco Seasoning
- two tbsps diced red onion
- two tbsps pimento or cherry pepper (halved lengthwise)

Directions:
1. Put one tbsp of cream cheese on one tortilla and top with taco seasoning.
2. Top with 1four teacups spinach, one tbsp red onion, one tbsp pimento pepper and 2 ounces roast meat.

Per serving: Calories: 278kcal; Carbs: 27g; Protein: 18g; Fat: 11g; Sodium: 116mg

55. Seafood Risotto

Preparation time: fifteen mins
Cooking time: thirty mins
Servings: four
Ingredients:

- six teacups vegetable broth
- three tbsps extra-virgin olive oil
- 3 pieces garlic (crushed)
- half tsp saffron threads
- one big onion (severed)
- one and half teacups arborio rice
- half tsps salt
- 8 ounces shrimp (21 to 25), skinned and deveined
- 8 ounces scallops

Directions:
1. Raise the broth to a simmer across low flame.
2. In a griddle, blend the rice with the salt and one teacup of the broth. Combine the components, then cook them blended across a low flame for a while, stirring occasionally, till the majority of the liquid is engrosses.
3. Repeat steps with broth, including half teacup of broth at a time, and cook till all but half teacup of the broth is engrossed.
4. Include the shrimp and scallops when you stir in the final half teacup of broth. Cover and let cook for ten mins. Serve warm.

Per serving: Calories: 460kcal; Carbs: 64g; Protein: 24g; Fat: 12g; Sodium: 430mg

56. Chicken & Goat Cheese Skillet

Preparation time: ten mins
Cooking time: ten mins
Servings: four
Ingredients:

- one lb. boneless, skinless chicken breast, cut into one-inch parts
- quarter tsp pepper
- two teacups 1-inch cut fresh asparagus
- 6 plum tomatoes, severed
- quarter teacup crumbled herbed fresh goat cheese +extra to serve
- half tsp salt
- four tsps olive oil
- two pieces garlic, crushed
- six tbsps low-fat milk
- Hot cooked rice or pasta to serve

Directions:

1. Put a pan on flame, include oil to it and let it heat. Sprinkle salt & pepper across the chicken then place in the pan.
2. Cook till it is not pink anymore. Eliminate the chicken and place it inside a container using a slotted spoon.
3. Keep it warm. Put asparagus in the similar pot and cook across moderate-high flame for a minute. Stir in garlic and cook till you get a nice aroma.
4. Include milk, tomatoes, and goat cheese and stir. Cover then cook for a couple of mins till the cheese melts. Include chicken and stir. To serve: Put one and half teacups chicken mixture on each of the 4 serving plates.
5. Put some hot cooked rice or pasta. Garnish with some more feta cheese, and serve.

Per serving: Calories: 524kcal; Carbs: 51g; Protein: 13g; Fat: 31g; Sodium: 525mg

57. Lamb Chops With Minted Peas And Feta

Preparation time: two hrs
Cooking time: one hr forty-five mins
Servings: two
Ingredients:

- 2 thick lamb loin chops around 6 ounces or 4 lamb cutlets
- one tsp olive oil. For the crushed peas and feta
- 8 ounces frozen peas
- one tbsp olive oil
- three tsps pine nuts toasted
- one red chili finely diced
- two tsps fresh mint leaves finely severed
- 3 tbsp feta

Directions:

1. Sauté the lamb on both sides with sea salt and powdered black pepper. Cook the chops for almost three to seven mins on each side, liable on thickness, or till done as required, on a grill, barbeque, or frying pot across moderate-high flame.
2. In the end, switch to the fat side for 30 seconds. In the meantime, fill a pan midway with water then raise it to a boil to create the minted peas. Cook for three mins once including the peas. Return the peas to the pan and lightly mash them.
3. Include the olive oil, pine nuts, and chili, then top with the mint and feta crumbles. Toss lightly with a generous amount of ground black pepper.
4. To serve, split the lamb and smashed peas between two plates.

Per serving: Calories: 286kcal; Carbs: 26g; Protein: 17g; Fat: 19g; Sodium: 289mg

58. Prawn Nasi Goreng

Preparation time: twenty mins
Cooking time: thirty-five mins
Servings: two
Ingredients:

- two tbsps coconut
- one average onion, skinned and diced
- one red pepper cut into roughly 1" chunks
- ½ small Savoy cabbage leaves finely cut
- two garlic pieces, skinned and finely cut
- four tsps root ginger, skinned and finely grated
- half–one tsp crushed dried chili flakes
- one and half teacups cauliflower rice
- two tbsps soya sauce
- 5 ounces prawns
- Generous handful of fresh coriander leaves roughly severed
- four tsps roasted peanuts, roughly severed

Directions:

1. Use a big nonstick frying pot or wok, and warm the oil across moderate-high flame. two–three mins, mixing regularly, stir-fry the onion, red pepper, and cabbage.
2. Stir in the garlic, ginger, chili, and cauliflower rice for another two–three mins, or till the cauliflower is heated through.
3. Cook for another one–two mins, swirling and tossing till the prawns are heated, prior to including the soy sauce, prawns, and half of the coriander if using. To taste:
4. Include extra soy sauce.
5. If using, top with the severed nuts and the leftover coriander, and split between bowls.

Per serving: Calories: 354kcal; Carbs: 23g; Protein: 21g; Fat: 17g; Sodium: 86mg

59. Steak Tuna

Preparation time: thirty-five mins
Cooking time: fifty mins
Servings: one
Ingredients:

- 4 oz. fresh tuna steak, cut into roughly 1" chunks
- one tbsp coconut or rapeseed oil
- 10-12 ounces pack of stir-fry vegetables
- two tbsps ready-made hoisin sauce
- Pinch crushed dried chili

Directions:

1. Sprinkle salt and black pepper on tuna. Warm the oil inside a huge nonstick frying pot or wok across high flame then stir fry the tuna and veggies for three–four mins, or till the tuna is gently browned, or according to the package directions.
2. Spray the hoisin sauce across the fish and veggies and toss for another 20– 30 seconds. If using, top with the chili flakes and serve instantly.

Per serving: Calories: 308kcal; Carbs: 16g; Protein: 31g; Fat: 13g; Sodium: 224mg

60. Pork and Sweet Potatoes

Preparation time: ten mins
Cooking time: one hr and twenty mins
Servings: 8
Ingredients:

- 2 pounds sweet potatoes, severed
- A spray of olive oil
- 1 yellow onion, severed
- 2 pounds pork meat, ground
- one tbsp chili powder
- Black pepper to the taste
- one tsp cumin, ground
- half tsp garlic powder

- half tsp oregano, severed
- half tsp cinnamon powder
- one teacup low-sodium veggie stock
- half teacup cilantro, severed

Directions:
1. Warm a pot with the oil across moderate-high flame, include sweet potatoes and onion, stir, cook for fifteen mins and transfer to a bowl.
2. Heat the pan again across moderate-high flame, include pork, stir and brown for five mins. Include black pepper, cumin, garlic powder, oregano, chili powder, and cinnamon, stock, return potatoes and onion, stir and cook for one hr across moderate flame.
3. Include the cilantro, toss, split into bowls and serve.

Per serving: Calories: 296kcal; Carbs: 26g; Protein: 11g; Fat: 8g; Sodium: 209mg

61. Lemon-Parsley Chicken Breast

Preparation time: fifteen mins
Cooking time: fifteen mins
Servings: two
Ingredients:

- 2 chicken breasts, skinless, boneless
- one-third teacup white wine
- one-third teacup lemon juice
- four garlic pieces, crushed
- three tbsps bread crumbs
- two tbsps flavorless oil (olive, canola, or sunflower)
- quarter teacup fresh parsley

Directions:
1. Mix the wine, lemon juice, plus garlic in a measuring cup. Pound each chicken breast till they are ¼ inch thick. Coat the chicken with bread crumbs, and warm the oil in a large griddle.
2. Fry the chicken within 6 minutes on each side till they turn brown. Stir in the wine mixture across the chicken. Simmer for five mins. Pour any extra juices across the chicken. Garnish with parsley.

Per serving: Calories: 117kcal; Carbs: 74g; Protein: 14g; Fat: 12g; Sodium: 189mg

62. Grilled Salmon With Papaya-Mint Salsa

Preparation time: ten mins
Cooking time: forty mins
Servings: four
Ingredients:

- 4 salmon steaks
- quarter teacup papaya
- quarter teacup bell pepper
- one tsp fresh ginger
- one tbsp pimiento
- one tbsp fresh mint
- one tbsp rice wine or white vinegar
- one tbsp fresh lime juice
- quarter teacup green onion
- one tsp jalapeño pepper
- Vegetable oil cooking spray

Directions:
1. Inside a container, include and mix all of the components for the salsa, except the salmon. Refrigerate round about thirty mins after covering.
2. Cooking Oil the grill or broiler pan lightly.
3. Sauté the salmon on both sides with pepper. five mins on each side on the grill or under the broiler, or till done. quarter teacup salsa on top of each salmon steak.

Per serving: Calories: 194kcal; Carbs: 3g; Protein: 25g; Fat: 8.9g; Sodium: 116mg

63. Pork and Pumpkin Chili
Preparation time: ten mins
Cooking time: one hr and thirty mins
Servings: 6
Ingredients:

- 1 green bell pepper, severed
- two teacups yellow onion, severed
- one tbsp olive oil
- 6 garlic pieces, crushed
- 28 ounces canned tomatoes, no-salt-included and severed
- ½ pounds pork, ground
- 6 ounces low-sodium tomato paste
- 14 ounces pumpkin puree
- one teacup low-sodium chicken stock
- two and half tsps oregano, dried
- one and half tsps cinnamon, ground
- one and half tbsps chili powder
- Black pepper to the taste

Directions:

1. Heat a pot with the oil on a moderate-high flame, include bell peppers and onion, stir and cook for seven mins. Include garlic and the pork, toss and cook for ten mins.
2. Include tomatoes, tomato paste, pumpkin puree, stock, oregano, cinnamon, chili powder and pepper, stir, cover, cook across moderate flame for one hr and ten mins, split into bowls and serve.

Per serving: Calories: 276kcal; Carbs: 36g; Protein: 11.5g; Fat: 10g; Sodium: 339mg

64. Pumpkin and Black Beans Chicken
Preparation time: fifteen mins
Cooking time: twenty-five mins
Servings: two
Ingredients:

- one tbsp essential olive oil
- one tbsp severed cilantro
- one teacup coconut milk
- 15 oz canned black beans, drained
- one lb. skinless and boneless chicken breasts
- two teacups water
- half teacup pumpkin flesh

Directions:

1. When using oil across moderate-high flame, heat a pan, include the chicken then cook for five mins.
2. Include the water, pumpkin, milk, and black beans, toss, cover the pan, diminish the heat and cook for twenty-five mins.
3. Include toss, cilantro, split between plates and serve. Enjoy!

Per serving: Calories: 254kcal; Carbs: 16g; Protein: 24g; Fat: 6g; Sodium: 92mg

65. Lemon Rosemary Branzino
Preparation time: fifteen mins
Cooking time: thirty mins
Servings: four
Ingredients:

- four tbsps extra-virgin olive oil, splited
- 2 (8-ounce) branzino fillets, preferably almost 1 inch thick
- 1 garlic clove, crushed
- half teacup sliced pitted kalamata or other good-quality black olives
- one big carrot, cut into ¼-inch rounds
- 10 to 12 small cherry tomatoes, halved
- half teacup dry white wine
- two tbsps paprika
- half tsps kosher salt

- ½ tablespoon ground chili pepper, preferably Turkish or Aleppo
- one small lemon, very finely cut

Directions:
1. Warm a large oven-safe sauté pan or griddle over high heat 'til hot, about two mins. Carefully include one tbsp of olive oil and heat till it shimmers, 10 to 15 seconds.
2. Brown, the Branzino fillets for two mins, skin-side up. Carefully flip the fillets skin-side down and cook for another two mins, till browned. Set aside.
3. Sprinkle 2 tbsp of olive oil around the griddle to coat evenly. Include the garlic, scallions, Kalamata olives, carrot, and tomatoes, and let the vegetables sauté for five mins till softened.
4. Include the wine, stirring till all components are well integrated. Carefully place the fish across the sauce.
5. While the oven is heating, brush the fillets with one tbsp of olive oil then season with paprika, salt, and chili pepper.
6. Top each fillet with the rosemary and the slices of lemon. Scatter the olives over fish and around the pan. Roast till lemon slices are browned or toasted for about ten mins.

Per serving: Calories: 201kcal; Carbs: 8.6g; Protein: 18g; Fat: 11g; Sodium: 815mg

66. Spicy Chicken with Minty Couscous

Preparation time: fifteen mins
Cooking time: twenty-five mins
Servings: two
Ingredients:

- 2 small chicken breasts, sliced
- one red chili pepper, finely severed
- 1 garlic clove, crushed
- 1 ginger root, 1" long skinned and grated
- one tsp ground cumin
- half tsp turmeric
- two tbsps extra-virgin olive oil
- 1 tweak sea salt
- three-quarter teacup couscous
- one small bunch of mint leaves (severed)
- 2 lemons, grate the rind and juice them

Directions:
1. Put the chicken breast slices and severed chili pepper in a large bowl. Sprinkle with crushed garlic, ginger, cumin, turmeric, and a tweak of salt. Include the grated rind of both lemons and the juice of 1 lemon. Pour one tablespoon of the olive oil across the chicken, coat evenly.
2. Cover the dish with a plastic wrapper and put in the fridge it within one hr. After one hr, coat a griddle with olive oil and fry the chicken. As the chicken is cooking, pour the couscous into a bowl and pour hot water over it, let it absorb the water (approximately five mins).
3. Fluff the couscous. Include some severed mint, the other tablespoon of olive oil, and juice from the second lemon. Top the couscous with the chicken. Garnish with severed mint. Serve immediately.

Per serving: Calories: 166kcal; Carbs: 52g; Protein: 106g; Fat: 17g; Sodium: 108mg

67. Mussels With Creamy Tarragon Sauce

Preparation time: twenty mins
Cooking time: twenty-five mins
Servings: two
Ingredients:

- 2 pounds fresh, live mussels

- one tbsp olive oil
- one average leek, trimmed and finely cut (around 4 oz. prepared weight)
- 2 garlic pieces, skinned and finely cut
- half teacup dry white wine
- 5 tablespoons full-Protein: crème fraiche
- 3–4 fresh tarragon stalks (around 1 tsp), leaves picked and roughly severed
- one tsp dried tarragon

Directions:
1. Eliminate the 'beards' by dumping the mussels into the sink and scrubbing them thoroughly under cold running water. Mussels with fractured shells or those that do not close when pounded on the sink's side should be discarded. Drain the ones that are good in a colander.
2. Warm the oil across low flame in a deep, lidded, wide-based saucepan or shallow casserole. Gently sauté the leek and garlic for two–three mins, or till softened but not browned.
3. Season generously with salt and pepper once including the white wine, crème Fraiche, and tarragon. Bring the wine to a simmer by increasing the heat under the pan. Cook for about four mins, or 'til most of the mussels have steamed open, after stirring in the mussels and covering closely with a lid.
4. Stir thoroughly, then cover and cook for another one–two mins, or 'til the rest of the vegetables are done.
5. Eliminate any mussels that haven't opened, split the mussels between two bowls, and pour the tarragon broth across the top.

Per serving: Calories: 381kcal; Carbs: 4g; Protein: 27g; Fat: 2g; Sodium: 236mg

68. Pesto Chicken Breasts

Preparation time: fifteen mins
Cooking time: ten mins
Servings: two
Ingredients:

- 4 medium boneless, skinless chicken breast halves
- one tbsp olive oil
- two tbsps homemade pesto
- two teacups finely severed zucchini
- two tbsps finely shredded asiago

Directions:
1. Cook your chicken in hot oil on medium heat within four mins in a large nonstick griddle. Flip the chicken, then put the zucchini.
2. Cook almost 5 to 8 more minutes or till the chicken is softened and no longer pink at a temperature of 170 deg. F, and squash is crisp, stirring squash gently. Disperse the pesto across the chicken and sprinkle with Asiago prior to serving.

Per serving: Calories: 230kcal; Carbs: 8g; Protein: 30g; Fat: 9g; Sodium: 578mg

69. Pork and Veggies Mix

Preparation time: fifteen mins
Cooking time: one hr
Servings: 6
Ingredients:

- 4 eggplants, cut into halves lengthwise
- 4 ounces olive oil
- 2 yellow onions, severed
- 4 ounces pork meat, ground
- 2 green bell peppers, severed
- one lb. tomatoes, severed
- 4 tomato slices
- two tbsps low-sodium tomato paste

- half teacup parsley, severed
- four garlic pieces, crushed
- half teacup hot water
- Black pepper to the taste

Directions:
1. First step is to heat the pan with the olive oil across moderate flame, place eggplant halves, cook for five mins and transfer to a plate.
2. Heat the pan across moderate flame, include onion, stir and cook for three mins.
3. Include bell peppers, pork, tomato paste, pepper, parsley and severed tomatoes, stir and cook for seven mins.
4. Arrange the eggplant halves in a baking tray, split garlic in each, spoon meat filling and top with a tomato slice.
5. Pour the water across them, across the tray with foil, bake in the oven and serve.

Per serving: Calories: 253kcal; Carbs: 12g; Protein: 16g; Fat: 3g; Sodium: 162mg

70. Spiced Up Pork Chops

Preparation time: four mins
Cooking time: fourteen mins
Servings: four
Ingredients:

- quarter teacup lime juice
- 1 Mango (sliced)
- 4 pork rib chops
- two tsps cumin
- one tbsp coconut oil (melted)
- 2 garlic pieces (skinned and crushed)
- one tbsp chili powder
- one tsp ground cinnamon
- quarter tsp salt and pepper as required
- half tsp hot pepper sauce

Directions:

1. Stir together lime juice, oil, garlic, cumin, cinnamon, chili powder, salt, pepper & hot pepper sauce inside a blending container. Then put in the pork chops.
2. Refrigerate for four hrs if kept on the side. Warm up your grill to medium and place the pork chops on it. Give seven mins for each side on the grill.
3. Serve with mango pieces, splited amongst serving dishes.

Per serving: Calories: 400kcal; Carbs: 3g; Protein: 35g; Fat: 8g; Sodium: 136mg

71. Herbed Butter Pork Chops

Preparation time: ten mins
Cooking time: twenty-five mins
Servings: two
Ingredients:

- one tbsp almond butter (splited)
- 2 boneless pork chops
- one tbsp olive oil
- quarter tsp salt and pepper as required
- one tbsp dried
- Italian seasoning as required

Directions:
1. Warm up the oven to 350 deg. F. Take out the pork chops from the pan and dry them with a paper towel.
2. After that, put them on a baking dish. Include salt, pepper, and Italian seasoning as per taste. Spray olive oil over pork chops and smear half tbsp of butter on each chop. Warm up the oven to about 350 deg. F and bake for twenty-five mins.
3. Put the pork chops on two plates and spray with the butter juice. Serve.

Per serving: Calories: 333kcal; Carbs: 1g; Protein: 31g; Fat: 23g; Sodium: 242mg

72. Pork With Dates Sauce

Preparation time: ten mins
Cooking time: forty mins
Servings: 6
Ingredients:

- one and half lbs. pork tenderloin
- two tbsps water
- one-third teacup dates, pitted
- quarter tsp onion powder
- quarter tsp smoked paprika
- two tbsps mustard
- quarter teacup coconut amino
- Black pepper to the taste

Directions:

1. Inside your mixing container, mix dates with water, coconut amino, mustard, paprika, pepper and onion powder and blend well.
2. Put pork tenderloin in a roasting pan, include the dates sauce, toss to coat very well, introduce everything in the oven at 400 degrees F, bake for forty mins, slice the meat, split it and the sauce between plates and serve.

Per serving: Calories: 332kcal; Carbs: 50g; Protein: 7.4g; Fat: 13.7g; Sodium: 226mg

73. Ground Beef and Bell Peppers

Preparation time: ten mins
Cooking time: ten mins
Servings: two
Ingredients:

- one teacup spinach (severed)
- 1 onion (severed)
- one tbsp coconut oil
- 0.5-pound ground beef
- one red bell pepper (diced)
- quarter tsp salt
- quarter tsp black pepper

Directions:

1. In a pan, blend the onion and coconut oil, and sauté across moderate-high flame till the onion is gently browned.
2. Include the spinach, salt, and ground meat after that.
3. Stir fry till everything is done. Meanwhile, remove all of the seeds from the interior of the red bell pepper.
4. After that, remove the mixture from the pan and spoon it into the bell pepper. Serve.

Per serving: Calories: 357kcal; Carbs: 7.89g; Protein: 31.68g; Fat: 19.61g; Sodium: 136mg

74. Cilantro Lemon Shrimp

Preparation time: twenty mins
Cooking time: five mins
Servings: four
Ingredients:

- one-third teacup lemon juice
- four garlic pieces
- one teacup fresh cilantro leaves
- half tsp ground coriander
- three tbsps extra-virgin olive oil
- 1 ½ pounds large shrimp
- one tsp salt

Directions:

1. Pulse the lemon juice, garlic, cilantro, coriander, olive oil, and salt 10 times inside a mixing container. Put the shrimp inside a container or plastic zip-top bag, pour in the cilantro marinade, and let sit for fifteen mins.
2. Warm up a griddle on high heat. Put the shrimp and marinade in the griddle. Cook the shrimp for three mins on each side. Serve warm.

Per serving: Calories: 180kcal; Carbs: 5g; Protein: 28g; Fat: 4g; Sodium: 250mg

75. Parsley Scallops

Preparation time: five mins
Cooking time: fifteen mins
Servings: two
Ingredients:

- 16 large sea scallops
- quarter tsp salt and pepper as required
- 8 tablespoons almond butter
- one and half tbsps olive oil
- 2 garlic pieces (crushed)

Directions:

1. Include the oil to a pot then heat it across moderate flame. Season the scallops with salt & pepper in the meanwhile.
2. When the oil is heated, sear the scallops for two mins on each side, then continue with the remaining scallops. When the scallops are done, take them from the pan then include the butter to melt.
3. Cook for fifteen mins once including the garlic. Return the scallops to the pan and coat them with the sauce.
4. Serve and have fun!

Per serving: Calories: 409kcal; Carbs: 13.36g; Protein: 34g; Fat: 24.91g; Sodium: 290mg

Chapter 4. Recipes for Salads and Sauces

76. Pork and Greens Salad

Preparation time: ten mins
Cooking time: fifteen mins
Servings: two
Ingredients:

- ¼ pound pork chops, boneless and cut into strips
- 2 ounces white mushrooms, sliced
- half teacup Italian dressing
- two teacups mixed salad greens
- 2 ounces jarred artichoke hearts, drained
- quarter tsp salt and pepper as required to the taste
- half teacup basil, severed
- one tbsp olive oil

Directions:

1. Warm a pot with the oil across moderate-high flame, include the pork and brown for five mins.
2. Include the mushrooms, stir and sauté for five mins more.
3. Include the dressing, artichokes, salad greens, salt, pepper, and basil, cook for four-five mins, split everything into bowls and serve.

Per serving: Calories: 235kcal; Carbs: 14g; Protein: 11g; Fat: 4g; Sodium: 182mg

77. Garlic Potato Salad

Preparation time: ten mins
Cooking time: twenty mins
Servings: 6
Ingredients:

- 6 medium potatoes
- 3 pieces garlic, crushed
- one teacup sliced scallions
- quarter teacup olive oil
- two tbsps unflavored rice vinegar
- two tsps severed fresh rosemary
- Freshly ground black pepper, as required

Directions:

1. Boil till fork soft but still firm, about twenty mins depending on size.
2. Drain the potatoes and put them aside to cool. Cut into bite-sized chunks once cool sufficient to handle.
3. Toss the diced potatoes, garlic, and scallions together in a mixing basin.
4. Blend the olive oil, vinegar, and rosemary. Whisk in freshly ground black pepper till thoroughly blended.
5. Mix thoroughly or cover and chill till serving.

Per serving: Calories: 204kcal; Carbs: 28g; Protein: 2g; Fat: 9g; Sodium: 6mg

78. Tomato-Basil Sauce

Preparation time: ten mins
Cooking time: twenty mins
Servings: four
Ingredients:

- two teacups diced tomatoes (fresh or canned)
- two pieces garlic, crushed
- two tbsps extra-virgin olive oil
- quarter teacup severed fresh basil leaves
- half tsp dried oregano
- quarter tsp salt and pepper as required

Directions:

1. In your saucepan, heat the olive oil across moderate flame.
2. Include the crushed garlic and sauté for one-two mins till fragrant.
3. Include the diced tomatoes, dried oregano, salt, and pepper.
4. Simmer for fifteen-twenty mins, mixing irregularly, 'til the sauce thickens mildly.
5. Stir in the severed basil leaves.
6. Eliminate from heat then let it cool mildly prior to serving.
7. Use as a topping for whole wheat pasta or grilled vegetables.

Per serving: Calories: 80kcal; Carbs: 5g; Protein: 1g; Fat: 6g; Sodium: 5mg

79. Tomato, Cucumber, and Basil Salad

Preparation time: ten mins
Cooking time: zero mins
Servings: four
Ingredients:

- 2 small/medium cucumbers
- 4 ripe medium tomatoes, quartered
- one small onion, finely cut
- quarter teacup severed fresh basil
- three tbsps red wine vinegar
- one tbsp olive oil
- one piece garlic, crushed
- quarter tsp freshly ground black pepper

Directions:

1. Split the cucumber and carefully scrape out all the seeds with a spoon.
2. Slice the cucumber halves and place them inside a container. Include the tomatoes, onion, and basil.
3. Put the remaining components into a small bowl and whisk well to blend.
4. Pour the dressing across the salad then mix it well. Put it into freezer for some time and serve it.

Per serving: Calories: 66kcal; Carbs: 8g; Protein: 1g; Fat: 4g; Sodium: 9mg

80. Warm Potato Salad with Spinach

Preparation time: ten mins
Cooking time: fifteen mins
Servings: 8
Ingredients:

- 3 pounds small new potatoes or fingerlings
- four teacups fresh baby spinach
- 5 tablespoons red wine vinegar
- 5 tablespoons olive oil
- two tbsps water
- one tbsp no-salt-included prepared mustard
- one tbsp agave nectar
- one tsp garlic powder
- one tsp all-purpose salt-free seasoning
- half tsp dried dill
- half tsp dried Italian seasoning
- half tsp dried thyme
- Freshly ground black pepper, as required

Directions:

1. Put unskinned potatoes into a pot and include sufficient water to cover by inches. Once boiling, diminish heat to medium to high and simmer till tender, about fifteen mins.
2. Eliminate pot from heat and drain. Cut the potatoes into bite-sized chunks.
3. Blend the other components in a dish, then pour so over salad. To coat and mix, whisk thoroughly.
4. Serve immediately or cover it and put in the fridge till ready to serve.

Per serving: Calories: 242kcal; Carbs: 37g; Protein: 4g; Fat: 9g; Sodium: 20mg

81. Chicken BBQ Salad

Preparation time: ten mins
Cooking time: one hr and thirty mins
Servings: one
Ingredients:

- one tsp soy sauce
- 4 boneless, skinless chicken breasts
- two tbsps cilantros
- two tbsps extra-virgin olive oil
- two pieces garlic
- one tbsp ginger, crushed
- 2 yellow peppers, large
- half tsp hot red chili pepper flakes
- five and half teacups mixed salad greens
- three tbsps rice vinegar

Directions:

1. Mince fresh cilantro.
2. Whisk together pepper flakes, garlic, ginger, cilantro, and half of the oil in a large bowl.
3. Include chicken breasts and coat well. Cover and put in the fridge for 30 min.
4. Cut peppers into quarters.
5. Over moderate-high flame, grill pepper till they start to blacken, for about fifteen min. Eliminate them to plate.
6. Grill chicken breasts for fifteen mins per side, till done.
7. Chop chicken and warm grilled peppers into ½ inch wide strips. Toss peppers and chicken with vinegar and oil.

Per serving: Calories: 171kcal; Carbs: 5g; Protein: 25g; Fat: 5g; Sodium: 31mg

82. Sweet Potato Salad with Maple Vinaigrette

Preparation time: ten mins
Cooking time: twenty mins
Servings: 6
Ingredients:

- 4 small/medium sweet potatoes
- 1 (15-ounce) can no-salt-included garbanzo beans
- 4 scallions, sliced
- 1 shallot, crushed
- two tbsps pure maple syrup
- two tbsps freshly squeezed lemon juice
- half tsps olive oil
- half tsp dry ground mustard
- quarter tsp freshly ground black pepper

Directions:

1. Put unskinned sweet potatoes into a pot and include water to cover by a couple of inches.
2. Over high heat, raise to a boil. Once it begins to boil, decrease the heat and include & continue to cook till the vegetables are soft, approximately twenty mins.
3. Eliminate pot from heat and drain. Put the sweet potatoes under cold running water till cool sufficient to handle, then peel and cut into 1-inch chunks.
4. Put sweet potatoes into a mixing bowl, along with the beans, scallions, and shallot.
5. Blend the other components in a dish, then sprinkle across the salad. Toss gently to coat.
6. Serve immediately or cover it and put in the fridge till ready to serve.

Per serving: Calories: 224kcal; Carbs: 42g; Protein: 7g; Fat: 3g; Sodium: 33mg

83. Zucchini-Ribbon Salad

Preparation time: ten mins
Cooking time: zero mins
Servings: 6
Ingredients:

- 2 medium zucchinis
- one tbsp sesame oil
- 2 medium yellow squash
- three tbsps low-sodium soy sauce
- one-eighth tsp red pepper flakes
- two tbsps rice wine vinegar
- quarter tsp sugar
- half tsp sesame seeds

Directions:

1. Peel the zucchini and squash into long ribbons.
2. Whisk together the remaining components in a huge mixing basin.
3. Toss in the zucchini and squash to blend thoroughly.
4. Season with freshly ground pepper as required.

Per serving: Calories: 50kcal; Carbs: 5g; Protein: 2g; Fat: 2.8g; Sodium: 272mg

84. Tart Apple Salad with Yogurt and Honey Dressing

Preparation time: ten mins
Cooking time: zero mins
Servings: 6
Ingredients:

- 2 tart green apples, diced
- one small bulb fennel, including stalk and fronds, severed
- one and half teacups seedless red grapes, halved
- two tbsps freshly squeezed lemon juice
- quarter teacup low-fat vanilla yogurt
- one tsp honey

Directions:

1. In a mixing basin, include all of the components and whisk well to incorporate.
2. Serve instantly, or chill till willing to serve.

Per serving: Calories: 70kcal; Carbs: 16g; Protein: 1g; Fat: 1g; Sodium: 26mg

85. Mexican Vegetable Salad

Preparation time: five mins
Cooking time: zero mins
Servings: 6
Ingredients:

- 2 medium tomatoes (seeded and severed)
- 1 cucumber (cut into bite-size chunks)
- 1 jalapeño (seeded and finely severed)
- half average red onion (severed)
- one average red bell pepper (cut into chunks)
- two big (11 to 12 inches) stalks of celery (severed)
- two tsps Tabasco
- 2 limes (juiced)
- two tbsps fresh cilantro
- two tbsps olive oil
- quarter tsp salt and pepper as required

Directions:

1. In a mixing bowl, blend the veggies.
2. Serve with severed cilantro on top.
3. The salad should be dressed with spicy sauce, lime juice, and olive oil.
4. Salt & pepper as required.
5. Chill prior to serving.

Per serving: Calories: 70kcal; Carbs: 7g; Protein: 1g; Fat: 4.8g; Sodium: 88mg

86. Fresh Herb Sauce

Preparation time: five mins
Cooking time: zero mins
Servings: four
Ingredients:

- one teacup fresh parsley, severed
- half teacup fresh basil leaves, severed
- two pieces garlic, crushed
- two tbsps lemon juice
- two tbsps extra-virgin olive oil
- quarter tsp salt and pepper as required

Directions:

1. In your bowl, blend the severed parsley, basil, crushed garlic, lemon juice, and olive oil.
2. Season with salt and pepper as required.
3. Mix well 'til all components are evenly blended.
4. Serve immediately over grilled chicken, fish, or roasted vegetables.

Per serving: Calories: 70kcal; Carbs: 3g; Protein: 1g; Fat: 7g; Sodium: 10mg

87. Spicy Avocado Sauce

Preparation time: ten mins
Cooking time: zero mins
Servings: 6
Ingredients:

- 2 ripe avocados, pitted and skinned
- quarter teacup plain Greek yogurt
- two tbsps lime juice
- one small jalapeno pepper, seeded and severed
- two pieces garlic, crushed
- two tbsps severed fresh cilantro
- quarter tsp salt and pepper as required

Directions:

1. In blender or food processor, blend the avocados, Greek yogurt, lime juice, jalapeno pepper, crushed garlic, and cilantro.
2. Blend till uniform and creamy.
3. Season with salt and pepper as required.
4. Serve as a dip for vegetables or as a sauce for grilled chicken or fish.

Per serving: Calories: 100kcal; Carbs: 6g; Protein: 2g; Fat: 9g; Sodium: 15mg

88. Egg Salad

Preparation time: twenty mins
Cooking time: fifteen mins
Servings: one
Ingredients:

- one and half teacups pre-packaged salad greens
- 1/8 cup mozzarella cheese
- one teacup sweet bell pepper of your choice, severed
- ¼ tsp. black pepper
- 1 tbsp. avocado, diced
- two big eggs
- three-quarter teacup tomato, severed
- ¼ tsp. salt
- 8 cups cold water, separated
- one tsp. thyme, crushed
- half teacup cucumber, sliced
- one tsp. olive oil

Directions:

1. Empty four teacups of the cold water into a stockpot with the eggs and turn the burner on.
2. When the water starts to bubble, set a timer for seven mins.

3. Meanwhile, scrub and chop the tomato, cucumber, avocado, and bell pepper and transfer to a salad dish.
4. After the timer has chimed, remove the hot water and empty the remaining four teacups of cold water on top of the eggs. Set aside for approximately five mins.
5. Peel the egg after cooling and dice into small sections and transfer to the dish.
6. Blend the salad greens and shredded mozzarella cheese to the salad dish and turn till integrated with the vegetables.
7. Dispense the olive oil across the dish and blend the crushed thyme, pepper, and salt till mixed well.
8. serve immediately and enjoy!

Per serving: Calories: 314kcal; Carbs: 36g; Protein: 22g; Fat: 21g; Sodium: 309mg

89. Chipotle Chicken Salad

Preparation time: five mins
Cooking time: zero mins
Servings: four
Ingredients:

- two teacups cooked chicken (shredded)
- one teacup celery (severed)
- two tbsps chipotle peppers in adobo sauce
- quarter teacup red onions (diced)
- quarter tsp sea salt
- half teacup light or homemade mayonnaise
- one-eighth tsp black pepper

Directions:

1. In a large mixing basin, blend all of the components. Mix thoroughly.

Per serving: Calories: 195kcal; Carbs: 5g; Protein: 21g; Fat: 9.8g; Sodium: 442mg

90. Eggplant Salad

Preparation time: ten mins
Cooking time: fifty mins
Servings: 3
Ingredients:

- 2 eggplants (skinned and sliced)
- 2 garlic pieces
- half teacup egg-free mayonnaise
- 2 green bell pepper (sliced and remove seeds)
- half teacup fresh parsley
- quarter tsp salt and pepper as required

Directions:

1. Warm up the oven to 480 deg. F.
2. After that, put the eggplants and bell pepper on a baking pan.
3. Bake the veggies for approximately thirty mins, flipping midway through.
4. Then, blend the cooked veggies with the other components in a mixing dish.
5. Mix thoroughly.
6. Serve.

Per serving: Calories: 196kcal; Carbs: 13.4g; Protein: 14.6g; Fat: 10.8g; Sodium: 156mg

91. Cilantro-Lime Sauce

Preparation time: five mins
Cooking time: zero mins
Servings: four
Ingredients:

- one teacup fresh cilantro leaves
- quarter teacup lime juice
- two tbsps low-sodium soy sauce
- one tbsp honey
- one piece garlic, crushed
- quarter tsp ground cumin
- quarter tsp salt and pepper as required

Directions:
1. In blender or food processor, blend the cilantro leaves, lime juice, low-sodium soy sauce, honey, crushed garlic, cumin, salt, and pepper.
2. Blend till uniform and well mixed.
3. Adjust the seasoning according as required.
4. Use as a marinade for grilled chicken, a dressing for salads, or a sauce for roasted vegetables.

Per serving: Calories: 30kcal; Carbs: 7g; Protein: 1g; Fat: 0g; Sodium: 90mg

92. Strawberry Spinach Salad
Preparation time: ten mins
Cooking time: zero mins
Servings: 6
Ingredients:

- three teacups fresh spinach or a 6-ounce package of pre-washed spinach
- one tbsp red wine vinegar
- one teacup fresh strawberries (finely sliced)
- one tbsp fresh lemon juice
- one-eighth tsp dry mustard
- two tbsps honey
- three tbsps olive oil

Directions:
1. The spinach leaves should be washed and dried.
2. Put in a dish and tear into bite-size pieces.
3. Strawberries, cut, and go on top of the spinach.
4. Blend the vinegar, lemon juice, honey, dry mustard, and oil in a separate bowl.
5. Dress the spinach and strawberries with the dressing.
6. Toss thoroughly and serve instantly.

Per serving: Calories: 95kcal; Carbs: 9g; Protein: 1g; Fat: 6.9g; Sodium: 13mg

93. Mandarin Salad
Preparation time: five mins
Cooking time: zero mins
Servings: four
Ingredients:
Salad:

- half teacup dried cherries
- four teacups leaf lettuce/spinach
- one teacup mandarin oranges (packed in water or juice)
- quarter teacup toasted almonds
- 3 to 5 strips of low-sodium bacon or turkey bacon (cooked and crumbled)
- 2 medium apples (sliced)

Dressing:

- two tbsps sugar substitute (Splenda, or can use sugar)
- two tbsps of water
- two tbsps apple cider vinegar
- two tbsps olive oil
- Pepper as required
- quarter tsp salt

Directions:
1. Toss the salad components together.
2. In a separate dish, blend the dressing components in the order stated.
3. Just prior to serving, toss the salad with the dressing.

Per serving: Calories: 295kcal; Carbs: 37g; Protein: 7g; Fat: 14.8g; Sodium: 245mg

94. Lemon-Dill Yogurt Sauce

Preparation time: five mins
Cooking time: zero mins
Servings: 6
Ingredients:

- one teacup plain Greek yogurt
- two tbsps fresh dill, severed
- one tbsp lemon juice
- one piece garlic, crushed
- quarter tsp salt and pepper as required

Directions:

1. Inside a container, blend the Greek yogurt, severed dill, lemon juice, and crushed garlic.
2. Season with salt and pepper as required.
3. Stir till well blended.
4. Serve as a dressing for salads, a sauce for grilled chicken/fish, or as a dip for raw vegetables.

Per serving: Calories: 40kcal; Carbs: 2g; Protein: 6g; Fat: 0g; Sodium: 25mg

95. Mayo-Less Tuna Salad

Preparation time: ten mins
Cooking time: zero mins
Servings: two
Ingredients:

- 5 ounces tuna, canned in water, drained
- one teacup cooked pasta
- one tbsp extra-virgin olive oil
- one tbsp red wine vinegar
- quarter teacup green onion, sliced
- two teacups arugula
- one tbsp parmesan cheese, shredded
- half tsp black pepper

Directions:

1. In a large bowl, toss tuna with vinegar, arugula, oil, onion, and cooked pasta.
2. Divide the dish between 2 plates equally.
3. Top with pepper and parmesan prior to serving.
4. Serve hot.

Per serving: Calories: 84kcal; Carbs: 2.4g; Protein: 2g; Fat: 7.9g; Sodium: 51mg

96. Tropical Chicken Salad

Preparation time: five mins
Cooking time: twenty mins
Servings: 6
Ingredients:

- one lb. boneless, skinless chicken breast
- two tbsps apple cider vinegar
- Juice of 1 freshly squeezed lime
- two tbsps olive oil
- quarter teacup severed fresh cilantro
- half tsp ground white pepper
- 1 ripe mango, diced
- one small red onion, diced
- one small bell pepper, diced
- 1 jalapeño pepper, crushed
- two pieces garlic, crushed
- one teacup cooked no-salt-includeed black beans

Directions:

1. Put chicken breast into a pot and include sufficient water to cover. Bring to a boil over high heat. Once boiling, diminish heat mildly, and continue boiling for about twenty mins, till fully cooked. Eliminate from heat, drain, then put away to cool.
2. Place the vinegar, lime juice, olive oil, cilantro, and white pepper into a small bowl & whisk well to blend.

3. Once the chicken is cool to touch, cut it into bite-sized pieces. Put into a mixing bowl & include the mango, onion, peppers, garlic, and beans.
4. Dish it and save it into freezer

Per serving: Calories: 194kcal; Carbs: 15g; Protein: 20g; Fat: 6g; Sodium: 52mg

97. Summer Corn Salad with Peppers and Avocado

Preparation time: ten mins
Cooking time: zero mins
Servings: 6
Ingredients:

- 2 half teacups corn kernels (3 cooked fresh cobs, or frozen and thawed)
- one average red bell pepper
- 1 ripe avocado
- 1 jalapeño pepper, crushed
- 1 scallion, finely cut
- one piece garlic, crushed
- Juice of 1 fresh lime
- two tbsps olive oil
- Freshly ground black pepper, as required

Directions:
1. If using freshly cooked corn, cut the kernels from the cob carefully using a very sharp knife. Put inside a blending container.
2. Core and dice the red pepper, then peel and dice the avocado. Include to the bowl, along with the jalapeño, sliced scallion (white and green parts), and crushed garlic.
3. Mix all together lemon zest and salt inside a small container and olive oil. Season as required with freshly ground black pepper.
4. The dish is ready serve it as soon as possible and enjoy

Per serving: Calories: 200kcal; Carbs: 19g; Protein: 2g; Fat: 12g; Sodium: 290mg

98. Roasted Corn & Edamame Salad

Preparation time: forty-five mins
Cooking time: fifteen mins
Servings: 6
Ingredients:

- 2 ears fresh corn, unhusked
- one and quarter teacups cooked corn kernels
- quarter teacup red onion (severed)
- quarter teacup red bell pepper (diced small)
- one tbsp light mayonnaise
- one tbsp fresh lemon juice
- one tbsp fresh cilantro (finely severed)
- one and half tsps ginger (finely severed or grated)
- half teacup edamame (shelled)
- one-eighth tsp salt
- one-eighth tsp black pepper

Directions:
1. Soak fresh corn for thirty mins in cold water.
2. Warm up the grill to high. Grill for ten to fifteen mins in the husk, flipping once.
3. Allow cooling prior to removing the husks.
4. Cut the corn off the cob and place it in a basin.
5. Blend the remaining components in your mixing bowl.
6. Refrigerate till ready to serve, covered in plastic wrap.

Per serving: Calories: 65kcal; Carbs: 10g; Protein: 3g; Fat: 2.0g; Sodium: 71mg

99. Balsamic Glaze

Preparation time: five mins
Cooking time: fifteen mins
Servings: four
Ingredients:

- one teacup balsamic vinegar
- one tbsp honey
- one tsp mustard
- quarter tsp salt and pepper as required

Directions:

1. In your small saucepan, blend the balsamic vinegar, honey, mustard, salt, and pepper.
2. Boil the mixture across moderate flame.
3. Lower the heat to low then simmer for about fifteen mins 'til the sauce thickens and coats the back of a spoon.
4. Stir occasionally to prevent burning.
5. Eliminate from heat and let it cool prior to using.
6. Spray over grilled chicken, roasted vegetables, or use as a glaze for baked salmon.

Per serving: Calories: 60kcal; Carbs: 14g; Protein: 0g; Fat: 0g; Sodium: 10mg

100. Simple Autumn Salad

Preparation time: ten mins
Cooking time: zero mins
Servings: four
Ingredients:

- one big head of red leaf lettuce
- 1 pear, finely cut
- ½ small red onion, finely cut
- one-third teacup severed walnuts
- two tbsps red or white balsamic vinegar
- two tbsps olive oil
- one piece garlic, crushed

Directions:

1. Wash the lettuce, pat dry, and then tear it into bite-sized pieces. Put inside a container with the sliced pear, onion, and walnuts. Set aside.
2. In a small bowl include the vinegar, oil, garlic and whisk well to blend. Serve immediately.

Per serving: Calories: 224kcal; Carbs: 25g; Protein: 3g; Fat: 14g; Sodium: 29mg

Chapter 5. Recipes for Snacks

101. Mango Salsa Wontons

Preparation time: five mins
Cooking time: fifteen mins
Servings: 24
Ingredients:

- Vegetable oil cooking spray
- one tbsp olive oil
- one big ripe mango
- one small cucumber
- half average red onion
- two to three tbsps fresh lime juice
- two to three tbsps severed
- Fresh cilantro
- 24 wonton sheets
- Pinch of cayenne pepper

Directions:

1. Warm up the oven to 350 deg. F.
2. Coat muffin pans with cooking spray and use wonton sheets to line the molds.
3. Warm up oven to 350 deg. F then bake for nine-twelve mins, or 'til golden brown.
4. Allow the wonton cups to cool. Toss in the other components, along with a tweak of black pepper as required.
5. Serve each wonton filled with salsa.

Per serving: Calories: 40kcal; Carbs: 7g; Protein: 1g; Fat: 0.7g; Sodium: 6mg

102. Cauliflower And Leeks

Preparation time: ten mins
Cooking time: twenty mins
Servings: four
Ingredients:

- one and half teacups leeks (severed)
- one and half teacups cauliflower florets
- one + half teacups artichoke hearts
- two tbsps coconut oil (melted)
- two garlic pieces (crushed)
- Black pepper as required

Directions:

1. Warm the oil in the griddle across moderate-high flame, then include the garlic, leeks, cauliflower florets, and artichoke hearts and simmer for twenty mins, mixing irregularly.
2. Stir in the black pepper, split across plates, and serve.

Per serving: Calories: 192kcal; Carbs: 35.1g; Protein: 5.1g; Fat: 6.9g; Sodium: 76mg

103. Sweet and Spicy Kettle Corn

Preparation time: 1 minute
Cooking time: five mins
Servings: 8
Ingredients:

- one teacup popcorn kernels
- three tbsps olive oil
- half teacup brown sugar
- Pinch cayenne pepper

Directions:

1. Include the olive oil and a few popcorn kernels to a big saucepan covering medium heat.
2. Lightly shake the saucepan till the popcorn kernels pop.
3. Toss in the remaining kernels as well as the sugar to the saucepan.
4. Shake the pot regularly while popping the kernels till they are all popped. Eliminate

the popcorn from the kettle and put it in a large mixing dish.
5. Serve the popcorn with a dash of cayenne pepper.

Per serving: Calories: 186kcal; Carbs: 30g; Protein: 3g; Fat: 6g; Sodium: 5mg

104. Eggplant And Mushroom Sauté
Preparation time: ten mins
Cooking time: thirty mins
Servings: four
Ingredients:

- 2 pounds oyster mushrooms (severed)
- 6 ounces shallots (skinned, severed)
- 3 celery stalks (severed)
- one yellow onion (severed)
- two eggplants (cubed)
- one tbsp parsley (severed)
- Black pepper as required
- one tbsp savory (dried)
- three tbsps coconut oil (dissolved)
- quarter tsp sea salt

Directions:
1. Warm the oil in a pot on a moderate-high flame, then include the onion, stir, and cook for four mins.
2. Stir in the shallots and simmer for additional four mins. Cook for fifteen mins once including the eggplant pieces, mushrooms, celery, savory, and black pepper as required.
3. Stir in the parsley, simmer for a couple of mins longer, then split across plates and serve.

Per serving: Calories: 101.3kcal; Carbs: 156.5g; Protein: 69.1g; Fat: 10.9g; Sodium: 105mg

105. Mexican Layer Dip
Preparation time: ten mins
Cooking time: zero mins
Servings: 15
Ingredients:

- one tbsp lemon juice
- A 15-ounce of can beans
- half teacup cream
- 3 avocados
- half teacup plum tomato
- half teacup of cheese
- one tbsp mayonnaise
- two tbsps fresh cilantro
- three tbsps taco seasoning
- half teacup diced onion
- 2 bell peppers
- two to three teacups lettuce

Directions:
1. Evenly put the components in a baking pan.
2. Refried black beans are the first layer. 2nd layer: mayonnaise, lemon juice, and mashed potatoes with ripe avocados.
3. Layer 3: Blend sour cream, cilantro, and diminished-sodium taco seasoning.
4. Peppers (bell) (layer 4) (layer 5) shredded cheese shredded lettuce (layer 6) 7th layer: diced plum tomato and onion.

Per serving: Calories: 110kcal; Carbs: 11g; Protein: 4g; Fat: 6.7g; Sodium: 130mg

106. Spicy Sweet Potatoes
Preparation time: ten mins
Cooking time: forty mins
Servings: four
Ingredients:

- 4 sweet potatoes (skinned and finely cut)
- two tsps nutmeg (ground)
- two tbsps coconut oil (melted)
- Cayenne pepper as required

Directions:
1. Toss sweet potato slices in a basin with nutmeg, cayenne, and oil to coat thoroughly.
2. Put them on a parchment-lined baking sheet then bake for twenty-five mins at 350 deg F.
3. Bake for another fifteen mins after flipping the potatoes, then split amongst plates and serve as a side dish.

Per serving: Calories: 242kcal; Carbs: 42.4g; Protein: 2.4g; Fat: 7.5g; Sodium: 75mg

107. Asparagus Bruschetta With Garlic And Basil

Preparation time: five mins
Cooking time: ten mins
Servings: two
Ingredients:

- one tbsp Olive oil
- one Ciabatta loaf or any other uncut small white loaf
- 4 Fresh asparagus spears (boiled till tender)
- ½ Garlic clove (crushed and finely severed)
- one tbsp basil (finely severed)

Directions:
1. Cut four 1" thick slices of bread from the loaf and set them on a baking pan, under a medium grill, lightly brown one side.
2. Cut the asparagus spears lengthwise in half and then into two or three shorter strips.
3. Blend the olive oil, garlic, and basil inside a container and distribute across the bread's untoasted side.
4. Return to the grill till the edges are browned, then top with asparagus and a light brushing of olive oil. While the dish is still hot, serve it instantly.

Per serving: Calories: 230kcal; Carbs: 13g; Protein: 8g; Fat: 8g; Sodium: 16mg

108. Hot Crab Dip

Preparation time: ten mins
Cooking time: twenty-five mins
Servings: 10
Ingredients:

- one package cheese
- one tbsp onion
- one-eighth tsp black pepper
- two tbsps creamer
- one cab crab meat
- one tsp lemon juice
- Cayenne pepper as required

Directions:
1. Warm up the oven to 375 deg. F.
2. Inside a mixing dish, soften the cream cheese.
3. Blend the onion, lemon juice, black pepper, and cayenne pepper in a huge mixing container.
4. Mix completely. Include the non-dairy creamer and mix thoroughly. Stir in the crab meat till everything is well blended.
5. Fill an oven-safe dish midway with the mixture.
6. Bake for fifteen mins, or 'til hot and bubbling, uncovered.

Per serving: Calories: 65kcal; Carbs: 3g; Protein: 5g; Fat: 3.7g; Sodium: 179mg

109. Mint Zucchini

Preparation time: ten mins
Cooking time: seven mins
Servings: four
Ingredients:

- two tbsps mint
- ½ tablespoon dill (severed)
- 2 zucchinis (halved lengthwise and then slice into half-moons)
- one tbsp coconut oil (melted)
- A tweak of cayenne pepper

Directions:
1. Warm the oil in your griddle on a moderate-high flame, include the zucchinis and cook for six mins, mixing irregularly.
2. Stir in the cayenne, dill, and mint, heat for another min, then split amongst plates and serve.

Per serving: Calories: 46kcal; Carbs: 3.5g; Protein: 1.3g; Fat: 3.6g; Sodium: 75mg

110. Sweet And Spicy Meatballs

Preparation time: ten mins
Cooking time: twenty-five mins
Servings: 18
Ingredients:

- Vegetable oil cooking spray
- quarter teacup onion
- one lb. ground beef
- one big egg white
- one-third teacup fine dry breadcrumbs
- quarter teacup fresh parsley
- one-eighth tsp nutmeg
- quarter teacup creamer
- half teacup cranberries
- half teacup grape jelly
- two tsps dry mustard
- one-eighth tsp cayenne pepper
- one tsp fresh lemon juice

Directions:
1. Warm up the oven to 375 deg. F.
2. Spray a small pot with cooking spray and set it on the stovetop on moderate-high flame.
3. Include the onion then cook till it is soft. In a mixing dish, blend the onion and the other 6 components.
4. Make 36 1-inch meatballs out of the mixture.
5. Cooking sprays a jelly roll pan or a small baking dish.
6. In a baking sheet, put the meatballs and bake for eighteen mins.
7. Meanwhile, make the sauce by mixing the cranberries and the sugar.
8. In your small saucepan, blend the rest of the components.
9. Cook across moderate flame till well heated. Pour the sauce across the meatballs on a serving dish.
10. Toothpicks are used to serve.

Per serving: Calories: 80kcal; Carbs: 8g; Protein: 5g; Fat: 2.9g; Sodium: 34mg

111. Broccoli And Almonds Mix

Preparation time: ten mins
Cooking time: eleven mins
Servings: four
Ingredients:

- one tbsp olive oil
- one lb. broccoli florets
- one garlic clove (crushed)
- one-third teacup almonds (severed)
- Black pepper as required

Directions:
1. Warm the oil in a pan on a moderate-high flame, include the almonds, toss to blend, and cook for five mins prior to transferring to a bowl.
2. Return the pan to moderate-high flame, then include the broccoli and garlic, stir, cover, and cook for another 6 mins. Stir in the almonds and season with black pepper as required, then split among plates and serve.

Per serving: Calories: 116kcal; Carbs: 9.5gm; Protein: 4.9g; Fat: 7.8g; Sodium: 75mg

112. Fresh Tzatziki
Preparation time: twenty mins
Cooking time: zero mins
Servings: 10
Ingredients:

- one big cucumber
- one tbsp lemon juice
- one teacup plain nonfat yogurt
- one tsp dried dill weed
- 4 large pieces of garlic
- quarter tsp salt

Directions:
1. In your mixing dish, blend the entire components.
2. Allow for a 20-minute rest period. Serve with cucumbers, broccoli, and carrots as a side dish.
3. Use as a salad dressing or a spread on a sandwich.
4. The leftovers will last 3 to 4 days in the refrigerator.

Per serving: Calories: 20kcal; Carbs: 3g; Protein: 2g; Fat: 0.1g; Sodium: 35mg

113. Squash And Cranberries
Preparation time: ten mins
Cooking time: thirty mins
Servings: two
Ingredients:

- one butternut squash (skinned and cubed)
- two garlic pieces (crushed)
- one small yellow onion (severed)
- one tbsp coconut oil
- 12 ounces coconut milk
- one tsp curry powder
- one tsp cinnamon powder
- half teacup cranberries

Directions:
1. Disperse squash pieces on a parchment-lined baking sheet, bake for fifteen mins at 425 deg. F, then put away.
2. Warm the oil in a pan on a moderate-high flame, then include the garlic & onion, constantly stirring for five mins.
3. Cook for three mins once including the roasted squash. Stir in the coconut milk, cranberries, cinnamon, and curry powder, and simmer for another five mins.
4. Serve as a side dish by dividing the mixture across plates.

Per serving: Calories: 518kcal; Carbs: 24.9g; Protein: 5.3g; Fat: 47.6g; Sodium: 70mg

114. Roasted Brussels Sprouts
Preparation time: ten mins
Cooking time: forty-five mins
Servings: 6
Ingredients:

- one lb. brussels sprout
- two tbsps olive oil
- one tbsp garlic
- one tsp fresh lemon juice

- Black pepper per taste
- half tsp salt
- quarter teacup cheese

Directions:
1. Warm up the oven to 350 deg. F. In a frying pot or a roasting pan, place Brussels sprouts.
2. Include the garlic and mix well. Lemon juice should be sprayed over Brussels sprouts. Toss the sprouts in the oil 'til they are fully covered.
3. Season with a sufficient amount of salt (almost half tsp) and a few grinds of black pepper.
4. Cook for twenty mins on the top shelf of the oven, then toss to coat Brussels sprouts with the oil in the pan.
5. Cook for a further ten minutes. Cook for another five mins once including the Parmesan (if using).
6. Warm the dish prior to serving.

Per serving: Calories: 85kcal; Carbs: 6g; Protein: 4g; Fat: 6.1g; Sodium: 128mg

115. Dill Carrots

Preparation time: ten mins
Cooking time: thirty mins
Servings: four
Ingredients:

- one lb. baby carrots
- one tbsp coconut oil (melted)
- two tbsps dill (severed)
- one tbsp coconut sugar
- A tweak of black pepper

Directions:
1. Inside a big saucepot, blend the carrots and sufficient water to cover them.
2. Raise to a boil on a moderate-high flame, then cover and cook for thirty mins.
3. Drain the carrots, place them in a mixing dish, and whisk the melted oil, black pepper, dill, and coconut sugar till well blended.
4. Split between plates and serve.

Per serving: Calories: 85kcal; Carbs: 13.4g; Protein: 1g; Fat: 3.6g; Sodium: 65mg

116. Spicy Kale Chips

Preparation time: twenty mins
Cooking time: twenty-five mins
Servings: six
Ingredients:

- two teacups kale
- two tsps olive oil
- quarter tsp chili powder
- Pinch cayenne pepper

Directions:
1. Warm up the oven to 300 deg. F. Set aside 2 baking sheets lined with parchment paper. Take the kale stems prior to tearing the leaves into 2-inch pieces.
2. Wash and dry the kale well. Spray olive oil across the kale in a huge mixing basin.
3. Toss the kale with the oil with your hands, ensuring each leaf is well coated. Toss the kale with chili powder and cayenne pepper to blend completely.
4. On each baking sheet, disperse the seasoned kale in a single layer. Make sure the leaves aren't overlapping. Bake the kale for twenty to twenty-five mins, flipping the pans once or till crisp and dry.
5. Eliminate the pots from the oven then let the chips cool for five mins on the trays. Serve instantly.

Per serving: Calories: 24kcal; Carbs: 2g; Protein: 1gm; Fat: 2gm; Sodium: 13mg

117. Cheese Herb Dip

Preparation time: twenty mins
Cooking time: zero mins
Servings: 8
Ingredients:

- one teacup cream cheese
- one tsp crushed garlic
- ½ scallion (green part only, finely severed)
- one tbsp severed fresh parsley
- one tbsp severed fresh basil
- half teacup unsweetened rice milk
- one tbsp freshly squeezed lemon juice
- half tsp severed fresh thyme
- quarter tsp freshly ground black pepper

Directions:

1. Blend the cream cheese, milk, scallion, parsley, basil, lemon juice, garlic, thyme, and pepper in a medium mixing container.
2. Refrigerate the dip for up to one 1 in a sealed container.

Per serving: Calories: 108kcal; Carbs: 3gm; Protein: 2gm; Fat: 10g; Sodium: 112mg

118. Cinnamon Tortillas Chips

Preparation time: fifteen mins
Cooking time: ten mins
Servings: 6
Ingredients:

- two tsps granulated sugar
- half tsp ground cinnamon
- 3 (6-inch) flour tortillas
- Cooking spray (for coating the tortillas)
- Pinch ground nutmeg

Directions:

1. Warm up the oven to 350 deg. F. Using parchment paper, line a baking sheet. Blend the sugar, cinnamon, & nutmeg inside a small container.
2. Spray both sides of the tortillas with cooking spray then place them in a clean work area. Using a pastry brush, evenly coat both sides of each tortilla with cinnamon sugar.
3. Put the tortillas on the baking sheet, cut into 16 wedges each. Bake the tortilla wedges for approximately ten mins, rotating once or till crisp.
4. Cool the chips completely prior to storing them in a sealed jar at room temp. for up to a week.

Per serving: Calories: 51kcal; Carbs: 9g; Protein: 1gm; Fat: 1gm; Sodium: 103mg

119. Grilled Sweet Potatoes And Scallions

Preparation time: ten mins
Cooking time: fifteen mins
Servings: four

Ingredients:

- four potatoes
- two tbsps Dijon mustard
- 8 medium scallions
- two tsps honey
- three-quarter teacup olive oil
- half teacup apple cider vinegar
- quarter teacup balsamic vinegar
- Freshly ground pepper as required
- quarter teacup parsley

Directions:

1. Warm up the grill to medium-high.
2. Brush the potatoes and onions with oil prior to placing them on the grill. three to four mins each side on the grill, or till potatoes are just tender.

3. Scallions should be grilled till tender and marked. Eliminate the scallions from the grill and slice them thinly. Blend half teacup olive oil, mustard, tablespoons of vinegar, and honey in a large mixing basin.
4. To taste, season with pepper.
5. Toss in the potatoes, scallions, and parsley till well coated.
6. Serve immediately on a plate.

Per serving: Calories: 570kcal; Carbs: 46g; Protein: 5g; Fat: 41.3g; Sodium: 257mg

120. Grilled Asparagus With Mozzarella

Preparation time: five mins
Cooking time: ten mins
Servings: four
Ingredients:
Asparagus:

- 20 asparagus stalks
- ¼ pound mozzarella

Dressing:

- four tbsps fresh lemon juice
- quarter teacup olive oil
- one tsp dried oregano
- one small shallot
- one tbsp fresh parsley
- Freshly ground pepper as required

Directions:
1. Warm up the grill to high. Mix all of the dressing components inside a small dish and put away.
2. Season asparagus with pepper as required after brushing with olive oil mixture. three–four mins on the grill, or till just tender.
3. Distribute the asparagus among four dishes and top with a piece of mozzarella right away.

Per serving: Calories: 230kcal; Carbs: 7gm; Protein: 10g; Fat: 19.5g; Sodium: 200mg

121. Celery And Kale Mix

Preparation time: ten mins
Cooking time: twenty mins
Servings: four
Ingredients:

- 2 celery stalks (severed)
- one tbsp coconut oil (melted)
- one small red bell pepper (severed)
- three tbsps water
- 5 cups kale (torn)

Directions:
1. Warm the oil in a griddle on a moderate-high flame, include the celery, stir, and cook for ten mins.
2. Cook for another ten mins once including the kale, water, and bell pepper.
3. Serve by dividing the mixture across plates.

Per serving: Calories: 81kcal; Carbs: 11.3g; Protein: 2.9g; Fat: 3.5g; Sodium: 75mg

122. Five Spice Chicken Lettuce Wraps

Preparation time: thirty mins
Cooking time: zero mins
Servings: eight
Ingredients:

- 6 ounces chicken breast
- 1 scallion
- ½ red apple
- ¼ English cucumber
- Juice of one lime
- Zest of one lime

- half teacup bean sprouts
- two tbsps Cilantro
- half tsp spice powder
- 8 Boston lettuce leaves

Directions:
1. Blend the chicken, sprouts, cucumber, cilantro, and other components and five-spice powder in a large mixing container.
2. Evenly distribute the chicken mixture among the 8 lettuce leaves.
3. Serve the lettuce wrapped around the chicken mixture.

Per serving: Calories: 51kcal; Carbs: 2g; Protein: 7gm; Fat: 2gm; Sodium: 16mg

123. Warm Potato And Kale Mix

Preparation time: ten mins
Cooking time: eighteen mins
Servings: two
Ingredients:

- two big potatoes
- one teacup fresh kale leaves
- half teacup onion
- one piece garlic
- one small tomato
- half tsp dried thyme
- half teacup beans
- one tbsp olive oil
- Pepper as required

Directions:
1. Potatoes should be diced and steamed till just tender (around ten mins). Eliminate from the equation.
2. Kale should be washed and stems removed prior to being cut into half-inch parts. Warm the oil in your nonstick griddle across moderate flame. Sauté the onion, garlic, and thyme till the onion is soft (around three mins).
3. Include the kale and tomato and cook for another one-two mins, or till the kale has wilted. Stir in the potatoes and beans till everything is well blended and heated.
4. Season with salt & pepper as required, then serve right away.

Per serving: Calories: 350kcal; Carbs: 65g; Protein: 10g; Fat: 7.4g; Sodium: 162mg

124. Kale, Mushrooms, And Red Chard Mix

Preparation time: ten mins
Cooking time: seventeen mins
Servings: four
Ingredients:

- ½ pound brown mushrooms (sliced)
- 5 cups kale (roughly severed)
- three teacups red chard (severed)
- one and half tbsps coconut oil
- two tbsps water
- Black pepper as required

Directions:
1. Warm the oil in a griddle on a moderate-high flame, include the mushrooms, stir, and cook for five mins.
2. Cook for ten mins once including red chard, kale, and water.
3. Toss in a tweak of black pepper, stir and simmer for another two mins.
4. Serve by dividing the mixture across plates.

Per serving: Calories: 97kcal; Carbs: 13.3g; Protein: 5.4g; Fat: 3.4g; Sodium: 79mg

125. Grilled Vegetables

Preparation time: five mins
Cooking time: twenty-five mins
Servings: four
Ingredients:

- one average onion (cut into large chunks)
- one average zucchini (cut into thick slices)
- two tbsps olive oil
- one average yellow squash (cut into thick slices)
- one small sweet potato (cut into small cubes)
- one clove garlic (crushed)
- quarter tsp salt
- Pepper as required

Directions:

1. In a large mixing basin, blend all of the veggies. Blend the oil, garlic, salt, and pepper; pour over the veggies.
2. Stir to coat all of the veggies. Arrange veggies in a grill basket or on a flat baking sheet.
3. Cook on a moderate-high grill for ten-twenty mins, or till the veggies are cooked and beginning to brown.
4. Serve right away.

Per serving: Calories: 80kcal; Carbs: 11g; Protein: 2gm; Fat: 3.9g; Sodium: 45mg

Chapter 6. Recipes for Cakes and Desserts

126. Stone Cobbler

Preparation time: fifteen mins
Cooking time: one hr
Servings: eight
Ingredients:

- quarter teacup packed brown sugar
- quarter teacup water
- two teacups rolled oats
- quarter teacup buttermilk
- two teacups peaches
- 5 tablespoon unsalted butter
- one tsp cinnamon
- one tsp baking powder
- two tbsps sugar
- two tbsps freshly squeezed lemon juice
- one and half teacups mildly undercooked quinoa
- quarter tsp grated nutmeg
- one tsp vanilla
- Cooking spray

Directions:

1. Warm up the oven to 350 deg. F. Spray the 9" x 13" baking dish with cooking spray.
2. Blend the peaches, lemon juice & brown sugar in a mixing basin. Set aside ten mins. Blend the sugar, oats, butter, baking powder, nutmeg, and cinnamon in a separate, large mixing dish.
3. Before the items create a gritty combination, work with your hands on them.
4. Blend the vanilla and buttermilk inside a blending container. Before a dough forms, blend all of the components. Disperse the quinoa uniformly over the lower part of the baking container.
5. Arrange the peaches and the peach juice over quinoa in the prepared dish. Scatter the dough over the fruit. Click down lightly.
6. For about thirty mins, bake till the dough is gently browned and the fruit is juicy and bubbling.
7. Warm it up prior to serving.

Per serving: Calories: 1004.35kcal; Carbs: 180.42g; Protein: 33.78g; Fat: 18.74g; Sodium: 295.18mg

127. Banana Cookies

Preparation time: ten mins
Cooking time: fifteen mins
Servings: four
Ingredients:

- one teacup almond butter
- quarter teacup stevia
- one tsp. vanilla extract
- two bananas, skinned and mashed
- one teacup gluten-free oats
- one tsp. cinnamon powder
- one teacup almonds, severed
- half teacup raisins

Directions:

1. Blend the butter with the stevia and the other components inside a container and mix well with a hand mixer.
2. Pour medium molds of this mixture onto a baking sheet lined with parchment paper then flatten mildly.

3. Bake the cookies at 325 deg. F for fifteen mins and serve them for breakfast.

Per serving: Calories: 280kcal; Carbs: 29g; Protein: 8g; Fat: 16g; Sodium: 20mg

128. Apple Crunch Pie

Preparation time: ten mins
Cooking time: thirty-five mins
Servings: 6
Ingredients:

- one teacup of sugar
- 4 large tart apples (skinned, seeded and sliced)
- half teacup of all-purpose white flour
- one-third teacup margarine
- three-quarter teacup of rolled oat flakes
- half tsp of ground nutmeg

Directions:

1. Warm up the oven to 375 deg. F. Put the apples in a square pan that has been gently oiled (around 7 inches).
2. Blend the other components in an average mixing container and spread the batter over the apples.
3. Bake for thirty to thirty-five mins, or 'til golden brown on the top crust. Serve immediately.

Per serving: Calories: 261.9kcal; Carbs: 47.2g; Protein: 1.5g; Fat: 8g; Sodium: 81mg

129. Healthy Protein Bars

Preparation time: ten mins
Cooking time: ten mins
Servings: 10
Ingredients:

- 2 scoops of vanilla protein powder
- quarter teacup coconut oil (melted)
- one teacup almond butter
- one tsp cinnamon
- 18 drops of liquid Stevia
- quarter tsp salt

Directions:

1. Set aside a baking pan that has been sprayed with a cooking spray.
2. Blend eggs, butter, and peanut butter in a mixing dish and whisk 'til uniform.
3. Stir in the dry components 'til a uniform mixture form.
4. Bring the batter into the prepared baking pan then uniform it out evenly.
5. Warm up the oven to 350 deg. F then bake for thirty mins.
6. Cut into slices and serve.

Per serving: Calories: 190kcal; Carbs: 3.9g; Protein: 5.1g; Fat: 18g; Sodium: 105mg

130. Strawberry Pie

Preparation time: five mins
Cooking time: twenty-five mins
Servings: six
Ingredients:

- one unbaked (9 inches) pie shell
- four teacups strawberries
- two tbsps lemon juice
- one teacup of brown Swerve
- three tbsps arrowroot powder
- four-six tbsps whipped cream topping

Directions:

1. In a pie pan, spread the pie shell and bake it till golden brown.
2. In your mixing bowl, mix two teacups of strawberries, lemon juice, and arrowroot powder, and Swerve.
3. Inside a saucepot, boil the mixture across moderate flame 'til it thickens.

4. Let the filling to cool prior to spreading it into the pie crust.
5. The remaining strawberries should be sliced and put over the pie filling.
6. Refrigerate for one hr prior to serving with whipped cream as a garnish.
7. Enjoy while it's still hot.

Per serving: Calories: 236kcal; Carbs: 26g; Protein: 2.2g; Fat: 11.1g; Sodium: 2mg

131. Pineapple Meringues

Preparation time: ten mins
Cooking time: zero mins
Servings: four
Ingredients:

- four meringue nests
- 8 oz. crème fraîche
- 2 oz. stem ginger (severed)
- 8 oz. can of pineapple chunks

Directions:
1. On the serving dishes, arrange the meringue nests.
2. Blend the ginger, crème Fraiche, and pineapple pieces inside a blending container.
3. Over the meringue nests, pour the pineapple mixture. Serve.

Per serving: Calories: 312kcal; Carbs: 25g; Protein: 2.3g; Fat: 22.8g; Sodium: 23.1mg

132. Pound Cake with Pineapple

Preparation time: ten mins
Cooking time: fifty mins
Servings: 24
Ingredients:

- three teacups of all-purpose flour (sifted)
- three teacups of sugar
- 6 whole eggs + 3 egg whites
- one tsp of vanilla extract
- one and half teacups of butter
- 10 ounce can of pineapple chunks (washed and crushed, keep the juice aside)

For Glaze:

- one teacup of sugar
- 1 stick of unsalted butter or margarine
- Reserved juice from the pineapple

Directions:
1. Warm up the oven to 350 deg. F. Whisk the sugar and butter till uniform and creamy with a hand mixer.
2. Slowly pour in the eggs (one or two at a time) then whisk thoroughly after each addition. Include the vanilla extract, then the flour and whisk well.
3. Include the pineapple, which has been drained and diced. Fill a oild cake pan midway with the batter and bake for forty-five to fifty mins.
4. Blend the sugar, butter, and pineapple juice in a small pot. Bring to a boil, stirring every few seconds. Cook till the glaze has thickened to a creamy consistency.
5. While the cake is still hot, pour the glaze over it. Allow for almost 10 seconds of cooking time prior to serving.

Per serving: Calories: 407.4kcal; Carbs: 79g; Protein: 4.25g; Fat: 16.48g; Sodium: 118mg

133. Mint Banana Chocolate Sorbet

Preparation time: four hrs & five mins
Cooking time: zero mins
Servings: one
Ingredients:

- one frozen banana
- 2 to 3 tbsp. dark chocolate chips (60% cocoa or higher)
- 2 tbsp. crushed fresh mint

- 1 tbsp. almond butter
- 2 to 3 tbsp. goji (optional)

Directions:
1. Put the butter banana and mint inside a mixing container. Pulse to purée till creamy and uniform. Include the chocolate and goji, then pulse several more to blend well.
2. Pour the mixture inside a container or a ramekin, then freeze for almost four hrs prior to serving chilled.

Per serving: Calories: 291kcal; Carbs: 65g; Protein: 6g; Fat: 5g; Sodium: 31mg

134. Fudgesicles

Preparation time: fifteen mins
Cooking time: one hr
Servings: 8
Ingredients:

- one crushed chipotle pepper
- half teacup lite heavy cream
- two tbsps unsweetened cocoa
- quarter teacup brown sugar
- quarter tsp sea salt
- two teacups whole milk
- one tsp vanilla
- 6 oz. severed dark chocolate (semi-sweet)

Directions:
1. Put the cut chocolate in a big mixing cup. Blend the cream, milk, cocoa, sugar, and vanilla in a large pan across low flame. Bring to boil, then take it off the heat.
2. Pour a different kind of milk on top of the chocolate. Include a tweak of salt then set aside till the chocolate has melted. Inside a mixer, include the chipotle pepper and pulse till uniform.
3. Fill 8 ice pop molds or 3-ounce paper cups with the mixture if you don't have ice pop molds. one hr later, place spoons in the middle of paper cups.
4. Freeze for about 4-5 hours.

Per serving: Calories: 895.27kcal; Carbs: 91.53g; Protein: 16.92g; Fat: 52.98g; Sodium: 213.9mg

135. Simple Apple Compote

Preparation time: fifteen mins
Cooking time: ten mins
Servings: four
Ingredients:

- one tsp of cinnamon
- quarter teacup apple juice
- 6 apples (skinned, cored, and severed)
- quarter teacup raw honey

Directions:
1. Put the entire components in a stockpot. Stir to mix well, then cook across moderate-high flame for ten mins or till the apples are glazed by honey and lightly saucy. Stir constantly. Serve immediately.

Per serving: Calories: 46kcal; Carbs: 12.3g; Protein: 1.2g; Fat: 0.9g; Sodium: 1mg

136. Cocoa Fat Bombs

Preparation time: ten mins
Cooking time: five mins
Servings: 8
Ingredients:

- quarter teacup cocoa butter
- quarter teacup coconut oil
- half tsp vanilla
- 8 drops of liquid Stevia

Directions:
1. Dissolve the coconut oil & cocoa butter across low flame in a small saucepan.
2. Eliminate the pot from the heat.

3. Blend vanilla and Stevia inside a blending container.
4. Put the little silicone molds in the refrigerator till the mixture has been set.
5. Serve and have fun.

Per serving: Calories: 120kcal; Carbs: 0g; Protein: 0g; Fat: 13.6g; Sodium: 105mg

137. Light Pumpkin Pie Recipe

Preparation time: ten mins
Cooking time: zero mins
Servings: four
Ingredients:

- one lb. ginger slices
- 16 oz. pumpkin (packaged)
- half teacup egg whites
- one teacup sugar
- two tsps of pumpkin pie seasoning
- 12 oz. evaporated skim milk in a can

Directions:

1. Heat the oven to 350 deg. F. Inside a mixing container, grind the cookies. Spray a nine-inch glass pie pan lightly with veggie cooking spray. Evenly press the cookie crumbles into the pan.
2. Inside an average mixing basin, blend the remaining components. Fill into the crust and bake for forty-five mins, or 'til a knife immersed in the middle comes out clean.
3. Refrigerate any leftovers. Allow cooling prior to cutting into 8 wedges.

Per serving: Calories: 218kcal; Carbs: 26.21g; Protein: 5.2g; Fat: 10.9g; Sodium: 111mg

138. Stuffed Baked Apples

Preparation time: ten mins
Cooking time: ten mins
Servings: four
Ingredients:

- four golden Jonagold apples
- quarter teacup of flaked coconut
- quarter teacup of dried apricots, shredded
- half teacup of orange juice
- two tbsps of grated orange zest
- two tbsps brown sugar

Directions:

1. Trim the top third of the apples and use a knife to hollow out the center. Arrange in a microwave-safe baking dish, peeling ends up. Fill apple centers equally with a mixture of coconut, apricots, and orange zest.
2. Pour over apples a mixture of orange juice and brown sugar. Microwave on maximum for 7 to eight mins, or till apples are soft, carefully covered with vented plastic wrap. Allow cooling prior to serving.

Per serving: Calories: 168kcal; Carbs: 28g; Protein: 2g; Fat: 2.6g; Sodium: 4mg

139. Almond and Tahini Cookies

Preparation time: fifteen mins
Cooking time: twenty mins
Servings: four
Ingredients:

- one teacup of white flour, unbleached
- one teacup and two tbsps of complete wheat flour
- A third of a cup of almond meal
- half teacup of cold unadulterated butter, cut into chunks
- A third of a cup of sugar
- one tsp of extract de Vanille
- half tsp of salt
- two tsps of water
- ¼ + two tsps tahini paste

Directions:

1. Prepare and heat the oven to 350 deg. F. Line two baking pans with parchment paper.
2. In a food processor, meld plain white flour, wheat flour, almond meal, butter, sugar, vanilla, and salt. Process till the mixture resembles crumbles.
3. Process the water and tahini till a smooth dough form.
4. Pull the dough from the mixture and knead it on the counter a few times till it is smooth (if the dough feels very dry, dampen your hands then knead the dough mildly).
5. Make little dough balls, set them on the baking sheet, and gently flatten each one with your fingertips.
6. Heated the oven to 350 deg. F and bake for twelve-fourteen mins, or till golden brown.
7. Allow cooling fully prior to serving.

Per serving: Calories: 231kcal; Carbs: 21g; Protein: 6g; Fat: 14g; Sodium: 127mg

140. Peanut Butter and Chocolate Balls

Preparation time: forty-five mins
Cooking time: zero mins
Servings: 15 chocolate Balls
Ingredients:

- three-quarter teacup creamy peanut butter
- half tsp vanilla extract
- quarter teacup unsweetened cocoa powder
- two tbsps softened almond butter
- one and three-quarter teacups of maple sugar

Directions:

1. Warm up oven to 350 deg. F. Line a baking sheet with parchment paper. Inside a mixing dish, mix all of the components. Stir everything together well.
2. Divide the mixture into 12-15 parts, shape each part into a 1-inch ball, arrange the balls on the baking pan, put in the fridge for at least thirty mins, and then serve chilled.

Per serving: Calories: 146kcal; Carbs: 16.9g; Protein: 3.2g; Fat: 8.1g; Sodium: 43mg

141. Almond Bites

Preparation time: ten mins
Cooking time: ten mins
Servings: 12
Ingredients:

- half teacup almond meal
- two tbsps coconut butter
- 4 dates (pitted and severed)
- quarter teacup unsweetened chocolate chips
- one and half tsps vanilla

Directions:

1. Inside your mixing container, blend the dates then process for 30 seconds.
2. Process the other components, except the chocolate chips, till smooth. Process for 15 seconds once including the chocolate chips.
3. Form little balls out of the batter and set them on a baking sheet.
4. Refrigerate for one-two hrs prior to serving. Serve and have fun!

Per serving: Calories: 53kcal; Carbs: 4.2g; Protein: 1.1g; Fat: 3.8g; Sodium: 75mg

142. Baked Egg Custard

Preparation time: fifteen mins
Cooking time: thirty mins
Servings: four
Ingredients:

- 2 medium eggs (at room temperature)
- quarter teacup of semi-skimmed milk
- half tsp of nutmeg
- three tbsps of white sugar
- one tsp of vanilla extract

Directions:
1. Warm up the oven to 375 deg. F. Inside your blending container, combine the entire components then beat with a hand mixer for a few seconds or till creamy and homogeneous.
2. Pour the batter into gently oiled muffin pans.
3. Bake for twenty-five to thirty mins or 'til a knife immersed into the center comes out clean.

Per serving: Calories: 96.56kcal; Carbs: 10.5g; Protein: 3.5g; Fat: 2.91g; Sodium: 38mg

143. Walnut Oatmeal Chocolate Chip Cookie

Preparation time: fifteen mins
Cooking time: twenty mins
Servings: 6
Ingredients:

- two teacups oats, rolled (not quick-cooking).
- half teacup of flour (all-purpose)
- half teacup of pastry flour (whole wheat).
- one tsp of cinnamon powder
- Baking soda half teaspoon
- half of salt
- one tbsp of tahini
- four tbsps of unsalted cold butter, sliced thinly
- 2/3 cup of sugar, powdered
- 2/3 cup light brown sugar, packed
- A single huge egg
- one egg white
- one tbsp of extract de Vanille
- one teacup of chocolate chips, chocolate malt, or bittersweet
- half teacup of walnuts, crushed

Directions:
1. Prepare the oven to 350 deg. F then place racks in the top and bottom thirds. Use parchment paper or silicone liners to line two baking sheets.
2. Inside a container, include the entire components, including oats, wheat flour, cinnamon, baking soda, and salt.
3. Inside a big blending basin, use an electric mixer to combine the tahini and butter into a paste. Continue mixing powdered sugar and brown sugar till fully combined—the mixture will still be gritty.
4. Whisk the egg, egg white, and vanilla extract inside a new container.
5. Whisk in the oat combination with a wooden spoon till barely moistened.
6. Mix up the chocolate chips and walnuts inside a blending container.
7. Scoop one tbsp of the material into a ball with wet hands, lay on a lined baking sheet, and flatten till squat but not cracked.
8. Continue making flattened balls with the remaining batter, spacing them 2 inches apart.
9. Bake the cookies for 16 minutes, moving the pans from front to back and start to finish midway through.

10. Please leave it cool for five mins on the pans prior to fully putting it on a cooling rack.
11. Allow a couple of mins for the pans to cool prior to baking another batch.
12. Store for almost 2 days in a sealed container or freeze for extended storage.

Per serving: Calories: 161kcal; Carbs: 22g; Protein: 2.4g; Fat: 7.3g; Sodium: 110mg

144. Sweet Raspberry Candy

Preparation time: ten mins
Cooking time: five mins
Servings: twelve
Ingredients:

- half teacup dried raspberries
- three tbsps Swerve
- half teacup coconut oil
- 2 oz. cacao butter
- ½ tsp vanilla

Directions:

1. Dissolve the cacao butter & coconut oil together in a griddle across low flame. Remove the pan from the heat.
2. Inside a blending container, grind the raspberries. Stir vigorously to include the sugar and powdered raspberries in the combination of melted butter and coconut oil.
3. Put the little silicone candy molds in the refrigerator till the mixture has been set. Serve and have fun.

Per serving: Calories: 103kcal; Carbs: 1.1g; Protein: 0.1g; Fat: 11.5g; Sodium: 45mg

145. Raspberry Yogurt Basted Cantaloupe

Preparation time: fifteen mins
Cooking time: zero mins
Servings: 6
Ingredients:

- two teacups fresh raspberries, mashed
- one teacup plain coconut yogurt
- half tsp vanilla extract
- 1 cantaloupe, skinned and sliced
- half teacup toasted coconut flakes

Directions:

1. Blend the mashed raspberries with yogurt and vanilla extract inside a small container. Stir to mix thoroughly.
2. Put the cantaloupe slices on a platter, then top with the raspberry mixture and spread with toasted coconut. Serve instantly.

Per serving: Calories: 175kcal; Carbs: 10.9gm; Protein: 18g; Fat: 2gm; Sodium: 105mg

146. Dark Chocolate Trifle

Preparation time: ten mins
Cooking time: fifteen mins
Servings: four
Ingredients:

- one small plain sponge Swiss roll
- 3 oz. custard powder
- three tbsps sherry
- 5 oz. hot water
- 16 oz. canned mandarins
- 5 oz. double cream
- 2 cubes (dark chocolate, grated)

Directions:

1. Whisk the custard powder and water in a mixing basin till completely dissolved.
2. Mix the custard well inside a container till it turns creamy, then set aside for fifteen mins.
3. Cut the Swiss roll into four squares after spreading it out.

4. In each of the four serving glasses, place a Swiss roll. Mandarin, custard, cream, and chocolate are layered on the Swiss roll. Serve.

Per serving: Calories: 315kcal; Carbs: 40.1g; Protein: 2.9g; Fat: 13.5g; Sodium: 185mg

147. Rhubarb Cake

Preparation time: fifteen mins
Cooking time: one hr
Servings: sixteen
Ingredients:
For cake:

- 4 tablespoon unsalted butter
- 2 stalks rhubarb
- three-quarter teacup sugar
- one egg
- one teacup plain (low-fat yogurt)
- two teacups white flour
- one-eighth tsp salt
- one tsp baking soda

Topping:

- one-third teacup packed brown sugar
- one tsp cinnamon
- half teacup severed walnuts
- two tsps unsalted butter

Directions:

1. Warm up the oven to 350 deg. F. Spray an 8-inch square or circular baking sheet with cooking spray.
2. Put the sugar and butter in a mixing cup and whip with an immersion blender. In the container, crack the egg.
3. Before including the egg, a second time, whisk it well. Stir in the yogurt till it's completely smooth.
4. Cut the rhubarb into 1-inch pieces. Pour the starch, baking soda, and salt into a sieve and gently whisk them together in a basin.
5. Blend the dry components in the butter mixture. Apply the rhubarb to the mixture and mix thoroughly with a spoon. Put the batter in the baking dish and set it aside.
6. Blend the cinnamon, brown sugar, and nuts inside a small container to make the toppings. In a saucepan, melt the butter across low flame.
7. Pour heated butter over the cinnamon, sugar, and almonds into a mixing cup. Blend well with a wooden spoon.
8. Apply the almond topping evenly over the cake mix in a baking pan.
9. Bake 'til a toothpick introduced into the middle comes out clean.

Per serving: Calories: 1096.94kcal; Carbs: 158.13g; Protein: 24.4g; Fat: 43.44g; Sodium: 242.74mg

148. Baba Ghanoush

Preparation time: twenty mins
Cooking time: thirty mins
Servings: 6
Ingredients:

- one average eggplant (halved and scored with a crosshatch pattern on the cut sides)
- one tsp ground cumin
- one tbsp olive oil (plus extra for brushing)
- one tbsp lemon juice
- one big sweet onion (skinned and cubed)
- 2 garlic pieces (halved)
- one tsp ground coriander
- Freshly ground black pepper

Directions:
1. Warm up the oven to 400 deg. F. Warm up oven to 350 deg F. Line two baking pans with parchment paper.
2. Brush one baking sheet with olive oil and arrange the eggplant pieces cut-side down. Blend the onion, garlic, one tbsp olive oil, cumin, and coriander inside a small container.
3. On the second baking sheet, spread the seasoned onions.
4. Roast the onions for approximately twenty mins and the eggplant for thirty mins, or till softened and browned on both baking pans.
5. Scrape the eggplant flesh into a basin after removing the veggies from the oven. Toss the onions and garlic with the eggplant on a chopping board and roughly chop.
6. Include the lemon juice & pepper as required. Warm or cooled is fine.

Per serving: Calories: 45kcal; Carbs: 6g; Protein: 1g; Fat: 2g; Sodium: 3mg

149. Baked Custard

Preparation time: ten mins
Cooking time: thirty mins
Servings: one
Ingredients:

- half teacup low-fat milk
- one egg (beaten)
- one-eighth tsp nutmeg
- one-eighth tsp vanilla
- half teacup water
- Sweetener (as required)

Directions:
1. Warm the milk mildly in a pan prior to whisking in the egg, nutmeg, vanilla, and sugar.
2. Fill a ramekin midway with the custard mixture.
3. Put the ramekin in a baking pot and fill it midway with water.
4. Warm up the oven to 325 deg. F and bake the custard for thirty mins. Serve instantly.

Per serving: Calories: 127kcal; Carbs: 6.6g; Protein: 9.6g; Fat: 7g; Sodium: 3mg

150. Peanut Butter Fat Bombs

Preparation time: ten mins
Cooking time: ten mins
Servings: 12
Ingredients:

- four tbsps peanut butter
- two tbsps butter
- one and half tbsps cream cheese
- one tsp vanilla
- one tbsp swerve
- one tbsp unsweetened cocoa powder
- two tbsps coconut oil

Directions:
1. Microwave for 30 seconds after combining all ingredients on a microwave-safe plate.
2. Stir well prior to pouring into little silicone molds.
3. Put in the fridge till ready to use. Serve and have fun.

Per serving: Calories: 75kcal; Carbs: 2g; Protein: 2g; Fat: 7g; Sodium: 75mg

Chapter 7. BONUS: Diet Obstacles and Various Solutions

Maintaining a healthy diet can indeed be challenging, but there are several strategies and solutions to overcome common obstacles.

Meal Planning

Meal planning is an effective strategy for maintaining a healthy diet.

1. Set weekly time: Allocate a dedicated time each week to plan meals, considering your schedule and commitments.
2. Consider goals/preferences: Account for dietary goals, restrictions, and preferences to customize your meal plan.
3. Plan balanced meals: Include nutrient-rich foods from various groups in each meal.
4. Make a shopping list: Create a list based on planned meals to stay focused while grocery shopping.

Additional tips:

- Batch cooking: Prepare larger quantities for versatile use throughout the week.
- Utilize leftovers: Repurpose ingredients to minimize waste and save time.
- Keep it simple: Start with a few reliable recipes and gradually expand your options.
- Plan for snacks: Incorporate healthy snack options for between-meal hunger.

Healthy Alternatives

Making healthier substitutions and adding flavor to your meals can greatly enhance their nutritional value and taste. Here are some healthy alternatives and flavor-boosting options:

Dairy and Condiments:

- Swap sour cream/mayonnaise with Greek yogurt/avocado for creamy dips.
- Use low-fat/skim milk instead of whole milk.
- Try natural nut butter (almond/peanut) instead of sugary spreads.
- Pick mustard/hot sauce over high-sugar ketchup/BBQ sauce.

Grains and Breads:

- Choose whole-grain alternatives for white bread, pasta, and rice.
- Experiment with quinoa, bulgur, or brown rice.
- Wrap sandwiches with lettuce/collard greens instead of tortillas/bread.

Frying and Baking:

- Bake, grill, steam, or sauté instead of deep-frying.

- Use whole wheat or almond flour for breading.
- Make homemade baked sweet potato/zucchini fries.

Flavor Enhancers:

- Add herbs/spices like basil, cilantro, turmeric, cumin, garlic, ginger, or paprika.
- Use citrus juices/vinegar to brighten salads, marinades, and dressings.
- Include umami flavors with mushrooms, tomato paste, soy sauce, or miso paste.

Healthy Snack Swaps:

- Choose air-popped popcorn/kale chips instead of high-fat chips/crackers.
- Snack on fresh fruits/vegetables/trail mix (nuts and dried fruits) instead of sugary snacks.
- Opt for unsalted nuts/seeds over salted/flavored versions.

Preventing Hunger Attacks

1. **Eat balanced meals:** Include protein, healthy fats, and fiber in three main meals.
2. **Stay hydrated:** Drink water throughout the day to avoid mistaking thirst for hunger.
3. **Keep healthy snacks:** Have protein, fiber, or healthy fat-rich snacks on hand.
4. **Portion Control:** Use smaller plates, eat mindfully, and savor each bite.
5. **Recognize true hunger:** Assess if you're physically hungry or experiencing emotional cravings.
6. **Tune in to your body:** Eat when moderately hungry and stop when comfortably satisfied.

Reading Labels and Selecting Suitable Foods

1. Check ingredients for added sugars, unhealthy fats, and artificial additives. Choose products with shorter ingredient lists and recognizable ingredients.
2. Mind serving size and servings per container. Adjust nutritional information accordingly and consider the total nutritional value.
3. Read nutritional information for key nutrients. Compare values to dietary goals. Choose foods low in fats, sugars, and sodium, and high in fiber, vitamins, and minerals.
4. Understand %DV to assess how food fits into overall diet. Aim for lower %DV in saturated fat, sodium, and added sugars, and higher %DV in fiber, vitamins, and minerals.
5. Compare labels of similar products from different brands. Look for brands aligning with preferences for healthier ingredients and nutrient profiles.
6. Be cautious of marketing claims. Rely on ingredient list and nutritional information instead.

Organizing the Pantry

1. **Inventory and declutter:** Assess pantry, discard expired/unhealthy items to clear clutter for better organization.
2. **Categorize and group:** Create sections for grains, canned goods, snacks to group similar items together.

3. **Prioritize healthy staples:** Stock nutritious items like whole grains, canned beans, low-sodium broths/fruits/vegetables.
4. **Make healthy options visible:** Arrange pantry to highlight nutritious items at eye level, increasing likelihood of choosing them.
5. **Store unhealthy snacks wisely:** Keep processed foods in less accessible areas to reduce temptation.
6. **Use clear containers:** Opt for airtight, clear containers for grains, nuts, seeds, and dried fruits for freshness and easy identification.
7. **Label and date items:** Label containers or use transparent bins, date bulk purchases to track freshness.
1. Maintain regular checks: Assess pantry regularly, plan grocery shopping and meal prep accordingly.

Preparing Food in Advance
1. Set a specific time each week for food prep.
2. Plan meals and make a shopping list accordingly.
3. Cook larger quantities of certain foods for multiple meals.
4. Pre-cut and store vegetables for quick use.
5. Marinate meat in advance for time-saving and better flavors.
6. Portion and store meals for easy grab-and-go options.
7. Freeze meals and snacks for longer storage.
8. Label containers with name and date for freshness tracking.

Social and Emotional Obstacles
1. Share your dietary goals with friends and family to gain their support and make sticking to your goals easier.
2. Choose healthier restaurants or those with menus that cater to your dietary preferences when dining out. Prioritize grilled, baked, or steamed dishes over fried or heavily sauced ones. Plan your choices in advance by checking the menu.
3. Be mindful of your eating habits by listening to your hunger and fullness cues. Avoid using food to cope with emotional stress and find alternative activities like exercise, hobbies, or socializing to manage emotions.
4. Plan for social events by checking the menu or bringing a healthy dish to enjoy. This ensures suitable options are available and reduces the temptation for unhealthy choices.

30-Day Meal Plan

Days	Breakfast	Lunch	Dinner	Dessert
1	Breakfast Oatmeal	Spiced Winter Pork Roast	Spicy Chicken with Minty Couscous	Apple Crunch Pie
2	Chia Breakfast Pudding	Beef Stroganoff	Pesto Chicken Breasts	Mint Banana Chocolate Sorbet
3	Pumpkin Quinoa Porridge	Mediterranean Pork	Spiced Up Pork Chops	Light Pumpkin Pie Recipe
4	Breakfast Casserole	Chicken Divan	Ground Beef and Bell Peppers	Almond and Tahini Cookies
5	Slow Cooker French Toast Casserole	Balsamic-Roasted Chicken Breasts	Cilantro Lemon Shrimp	Baked Egg Custard
6	Maple Oatmeal	Sesame Chicken Veggie Wraps	Pumpkin and Black Beans Chicken	Sweet Raspberry Candy
7	Breakfast Tofu	Mediterranean Beef Dish	Pork and Sweet Potatoes	Rhubarb Cake
8	Ground Beef Breakfast Skillet	Mediterranean Fish Bake	Pork Strips and Rice	Baked Custard
9	Apple Cinnamon Steel Cut Oats	Shrimp with Garlic and Mushrooms	Fish with Peppers	Peanut Butter Fat Bombs
10	Breakfast Frittata	Pork with Scallions and Peanuts	Chicken & Goat Cheese Skillet	Pineapple Meringues
11	Triple Berry Steel Cut Oats	Ginger and Chili Baked Fish	Steak Tuna	Stone Cobbler
12	Tomato Omelet	Healthy, Juicy Salmon Dish	Lemon-Parsley Chicken Breast	Healthy Protein Bars
13	Breakfast Rice Porridge	Mussels with Tomatoes & Chili	Herbed Butter Pork Chops	Simple Apple Compote
14	Blueberry Low-Sodium Pancakes	Smoked Salmon Crudités	Parsley Scallops	Stuffed Baked Apples
15	Apples and Cinnamon Oatmeal	Sesame Salmon with Broccoli and Tomatoes	Mussels with Creamy Tarragon Sauce	Peanut Butter and Chocolate Balls
16	Breakfast Stuffed Biscuits	Chicken Veronique	Lemon Rosemary Branzino	Raspberry Yogurt Basted Cantaloupe
17	At-Home Cappuccino	Southwestern Chicken and Pasta	Prawn Nasi Goreng	Dark Chocolate Trifle
18	Gingerbread Oatmeal	Creamy Smoky Pork Chops	Seafood Risotto	Baba Ghanoush

19	Breakfast Eggnog	Thai Curry with Prawns	Taco-Seasoned Roast Beef Wraps	Almond Bites
20	Barley Porridge	Currant Pork Chops	Pork and Veggies Mix	Walnut Oatmeal Chocolate Chip Cookie
21	Banana Chia Pudding	Tuna and Potato Bake	Chicken Tomato and Green Beans	Strawberry Pie
22	Breakfast Omelet	Crunchy Fish Bites	Pork with Dates Sauce	Pound Cake with Pineapple
23	Apple Oats	Pork Chops and Apples	Lamb Chops with Minted Peas and Feta	Fudgesicles
24	Coconut Almond Granola	Baked Salmon	Pork and Pumpkin Chili	Banana Cookies
25	Breakfast Porridge	Chicken Chili	Grilled Salmon with Papaya-Mint Salsa	Cocoa Fat Bombs
26	Chia Breakfast Pudding	Sesame Chicken Veggie Wraps	Spicy Chicken with Minty Couscous	Sweet Raspberry Candy
27	Pumpkin Quinoa Porridge	Mediterranean Beef Dish	Pesto Chicken Breasts	Rhubarb Cake
28	Breakfast Casserole	Mediterranean Fish Bake	Lemon Rosemary Branzino	Baked Custard
29	Tomato Omelet	Healthy, Juicy Salmon Dish	Prawn Nasi Goreng	Mint Banana Chocolate Sorbet
30	Breakfast Rice Porridge	Mussels with Tomatoes & Chili	Seafood Risotto	Light Pumpkin Pie Recipe

In this book we provide you with a wide selection of 25 recipes for each category, including lunches, dinners, breakfasts, and snacks. This array of recipes gives you the freedom to personalize your dietary journey by selecting the combinations that suit you best.

In addition to the practical 30-day meal plan provided above we also suggest another method for creating your personalized meal plan. For example, you can independently choose 10 lunch recipes, 10 dinner recipes, 5 breakfast recipes, and 3 snack recipes, allowing you to create 1500 days of completely different recipes. This approach ensures that your Dash Diet remains varied and never repetitive, making it both enjoyable and sustainable in the long run. Use your creativity to generate practically infinite combinations. Experiment, explore, and develop a meal plan that aligns with your lifestyle and culinary preferences.

Measurement Conversion Chart

Volume Equivalents (Liquid)

US Standard	US Standard (ounces)	Metric (approximate)
two tbsps	1 fl. oz.	30 milliliter
quarter teacup	2 fl. oz.	60 milliliter
half teacup	4 fl. oz.	120 milliliter
one teacup	8 fl. oz.	240 milliliter
one and half teacups	12 fl. oz.	355 milliliter
two teacups or one pint	16 fl. oz.	475 milliliter
four teacups or one quart	32 fl. oz.	1 Liter
one gallon	128 fl. oz.	4 Liter

Volume Equivalents (Dry)

US Standard	Metric (approximate)
one-eighth tsp	0.5 milliliter
quarter tsp	1 milliliter
half tsp	2 milliliter
three-quarter tsp	4 milliliter
one tsp	5 milliliter
one tbsp	15 milliliter
quarter teacup	59 milliliter
one-third teacup	79 milliliter
half teacup	118 milliliter
two-third teacup	156 milliliter
three-quarter teacup	177 milliliter
one teacup	235 milliliter
two teacups or one pint	475 milliliter
three teacups	700 milliliter
four teacups or one quart	1 Liter

Oven Temperatures

Fahrenheit (F)	Celsius (C) (approximate)
250 degrees Fahrenheit	120 degrees Celsius
300 degrees Fahrenheit	150 degrees Celsius
325 degrees Fahrenheit	165 degrees Celsius
350 degrees Fahrenheit	180 degrees Celsius

375 degrees Fahrenheit	190 degrees Celsius
400 degrees Fahrenheit	200 degrees Celsius
425 degrees Fahrenheit	220 degrees Celsius
450 degrees Fahrenheit	230 degrees Celsius

Weight Equivalents

US Standard	Metric (approximate)
one tbsp	15 gm
half oz.	15 gm
one oz.	30 gm
two oz.	60 gm
four oz.	115 gm
eight oz.	225 gm
twelve oz.	340 gm
sixteen oz. or one lb.	455 gm

Recipe Index

Almond and Tahini Cookies; 71
Almond Bites; 72
Apple Cinnamon Steel Cut Oats; 18
Apple Crunch Pie; 68
Apple Oats; 23
Apples and Cinnamon Oatmeal; 23
Asparagus Bruschetta With Garlic And Basil; 59
At-Home Cappuccino; 22
Baba Ghanoush; 75
Baked Custard; 76
Baked Egg Custard; 73
Baked Salmon; 30
Balsamic Glaze; 56
Balsamic-Roasted Chicken Breasts; 34
Banana Chia Pudding; 21
Banana Cookies; 67
Barley Porridge; 22
Beef Stroganoff; 28
Blueberry Low-Sodium Pancakes; 22
Breakfast Casserole; 19
Breakfast Eggnog; 18
Breakfast Frittata; 23
Breakfast Oatmeal; 17
Breakfast Omelet; 16
Breakfast Porridge; 16
Breakfast Rice Porridge; 23
Breakfast Stuffed Biscuits; 19
Breakfast Tofu; 21
Broccoli And Almonds Mix; 60
Cauliflower And Leeks; 57
Celery And Kale Mix; 64
Cheese Herb Dip; 63
Chia Breakfast Pudding; 19
Chicken & Goat Cheese Skillet; 38
Chicken BBQ Salad; 49
Chicken Chili; 29
Chicken Divan; 33
Chicken Tomato and Green Beans; 36
Chicken Veronique; 28
Chipotle Chicken Salad; 52
Cilantro Lemon Shrimp; 45

Cilantro-Lime Sauce; 52
Cinnamon Tortillas Chips; 63
Cocoa Fat Bombs; 70
Coconut Almond Granola; 17
Creamy Smoky Pork Chops; 25
Crunchy Fish Bites; 33
Currant Pork Chops; 32
Dark Chocolate Trifle; 74
Dill Carrots; 62
Egg Salad; 51
Eggplant And Mushroom Sauté; 58
Eggplant Salad; 52
Fish with Peppers; 36
Five Spice Chicken Lettuce Wraps; 64
Fresh Herb Sauce; 51
Fresh Tzatziki; 61
Fudgesicles; 70
Garlic Potato Salad; 47
Ginger And Chili Baked Fish; 27
Gingerbread Oatmeal; 20
Grilled Asparagus With Mozzarella; 64
Grilled Salmon With Papaya-Mint Salsa; 40
Grilled Sweet Potatoes And Scallions; 63
Grilled Vegetables; 66
Ground Beef and Bell Peppers; 45
Ground Beef Breakfast Skillet; 19
Healthy Protein Bars; 68
Healthy, Juicy Salmon Dish; 30
Herbed Butter Pork Chops; 44
Hot Crab Dip; 59
Kale, Mushrooms, And Red Chard Mix; 65
Lamb Chops With Minted Peas And Feta; 38
Lemon Rosemary Branzino; 41
Lemon-Dill Yogurt Sauce; 54
Lemon-Parsley Chicken Breast; 40
Light Pumpkin Pie Recipe; 71
Mandarin Salad; 53
Mango Salsa Wontons; 57
Maple Oatmeal; 20
Mayo-Less Tuna Salad; 54
Mediterranean Beef Dish; 34

Mediterranean Fish Bake; 29
Mediterranean Pork; 31
Mexican Layer Dip; 58
Mexican Vegetable Salad; 50
Mint Banana Chocolate Sorbet; 69
Mint Zucchini; 60
Mussels With Creamy Tarragon Sauce; 42
Mussels with Tomatoes & Chili; 32
Parsley Scallops; 46
Peanut Butter and Chocolate Balls; 72
Peanut Butter Fat Bombs; 76
Pesto Chicken Breasts with Summer Squash; 43
Pineapple Meringues; 69
Pork and Greens Salad; 47
Pork and Pumpkin Chili; 41
Pork and Sweet Potatoes; 39
Pork and Veggies Mix; 43
Pork Chops And Apples; 26
Pork Strips and Rice; 36
Pork With Dates Sauce; 45
Pork with Scallions and Peanuts; 25
Pound Cake with Pineapple; 69
Prawn Nasi Goreng; 39
Pumpkin and Black Beans Chicken; 41
Pumpkin Quinoa Porridge; 20
Raspberry Yogurt Basted Cantaloupe; 74
Rhubarb Cake; 75
Roasted Brussels Sprouts; 61
Roasted Corn & Edamame Salad; 55
Seafood Risotto; 37
Sesame Chicken Veggie Wraps; 35
Sesame Salmon With Broccoli And Tomatoes; 31
Shrimp with Garlic and Mushrooms; 26
Simple Apple Compote; 70
Simple Autumn Salad; 56

Slow Cooker French Toast Casserole; 18
Smoked Salmon Crudités; 34
Southwestern Chicken and Pasta; 25
Spiced Up Pork Chops; 44
Spiced Winter Pork Roast; 26
Spicy Avocado Sauce; 51
Spicy Chicken with Minty Couscous; 42
Spicy Kale Chips; 62
Spicy Sweet Potatoes; 58
Squash And Cranberries; 61
Steak Tuna; 39
Stone Cobbler; 67
Strawberry Pie; 68
Strawberry Spinach Salad; 53
Stuffed Baked Apples; 71
Summer Corn Salad with Peppers and Avocado; 55
Sweet and Spicy Kettle Corn; 57
Sweet And Spicy Meatballs; 60
Sweet Potato Salad with Maple Vinaigrette; 49
Sweet Raspberry Candy; 74
Taco-Seasoned Roast Beef Wraps; 37
Tart Apple Salad with Yogurt and Honey Dressing; 50
Thai Curry with Prawns; 27
Tomato Omelet; 17
Tomato, Cucumber, and Basil Salad; 48
Tomato-Basil Sauce; 47
Triple Berry Steel Cut Oats; 16
Tropical Chicken Salad; 54
Tuna And Potato Bake; 32
Walnut Oatmeal Chocolate Chip Cookie; 73
Warm Potato And Kale Mix; 65
Warm Potato Salad with Spinach; 48
Zucchini-Ribbon Salad; 50

Conclusion

The Dash diet, known for its effectiveness in lowering blood pressure and sugar levels, is often abandoned by people due to limited dish options. However, this book provides a solution to this problem and can help individuals get back on track with the Dash diet. By following the Dash diet, you can experience various benefits such as feeling great, losing weight, and having more energy. The diet is also beneficial for ketosis, blood sugar control, and maintaining regularity. It is a simple and affordable approach to healthy eating that allows you to enjoy delicious foods without completely eliminating your favorites. Give the Dash diet a try and discover how easy it can be to embrace a healthy lifestyle.

Scientifically proven to be effective, the Dash diet has shown positive results in dropping the risk of heart attacks, strokes, heart failure, cancer, diabetic complications, and kidney stones. By emphasizing the consumption of a variety of foods while ensuring proper nutrient intake, the Dash diet promotes overall well-being. This unique cookbook provides a step-by-step process to help you embrace the Dash diet and develop a love for it. The recipes cater to all skill levels, from beginners to experts, making it accessible to everyone. With the cookbook's easy-to-follow instructions, you can effortlessly prepare meals that cover a range of caloric needs for breakfast, lunch, and dinner. This helps you stay organized and plan your meals in advance, considering the busy nature of our lives.

The meals recommended in the book not only align with the Dash diet principles but also offer delicious flavors and variety. By sticking to the diet and incorporating these recipes into your routine, you can expect to see noticeable results. Whether you prefer simple or intricate dishes, this cookbook has you covered and will turn you into a Dash diet expert in no time. It emphasizes that nutritious food doesn't have to be dull or tasteless, and provides recipes that are both enjoyable and healthy. If you're looking for an extensive selection of delicious recipes, this book is a perfect choice.

Thank you for taking the time to read and reflect the information provided. After reading this book, you will have a better understanding of the Dash diet and its benefits. Take the next step by gathering the necessary ingredients and experimenting with the recipes. Remember to complement the diet with regular exercise and a healthy lifestyle to maximize the results. Best of luck on your journey towards better health!

Made in the USA
Las Vegas, NV
30 November 2023